Zahra Ranjbar
Ommolbanin Az
Forough Ameri

Duties of Nurses in the ICU Special Care Unit

Zahra Ranjbar
Ommolbanin Az
Forough Ameri

Duties of Nurses in the ICU Special Care Unit

Noor Publishing

Imprint

Cover image: www.ingimage.com

Publisher:
Noor Publishing
is a trademark of
Dodo Books Indian Ocean Ltd., member of the OmniScriptum S.R.L Publishing group
str. A.Russo 15, of. 61, Chisinau-2068, Republic of Moldova Europe
Printed at: see last page
ISBN: 978-620-4-71975-7

Duties of Nurses in the ICU Special Care Unit

By

Zahra Ranjbar

Bachelor of Science in Anesthesia, Masters Student in Anesthesia Education at Ahvaz Jundishapur University of Medical Sciences, Iran

Ommolbanin Az

Nursing Expert, Third Rank in 2013, Graduated from Larestan University, Fars, Iran

Forough Ameri

Anesthesiology Resident at Iran University of Medical Science, Tehran, Iran

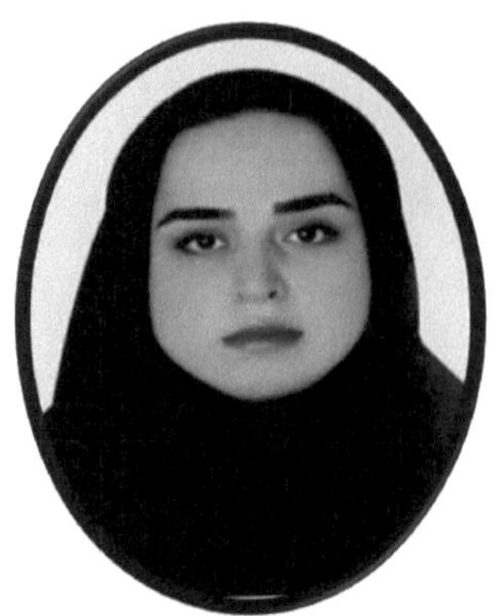

Zahra Ranjbar

Bachelor of Science in Anesthesia, Masters Student in Anesthesia Education at Ahvaz Jundishapur University of Medical Sciences

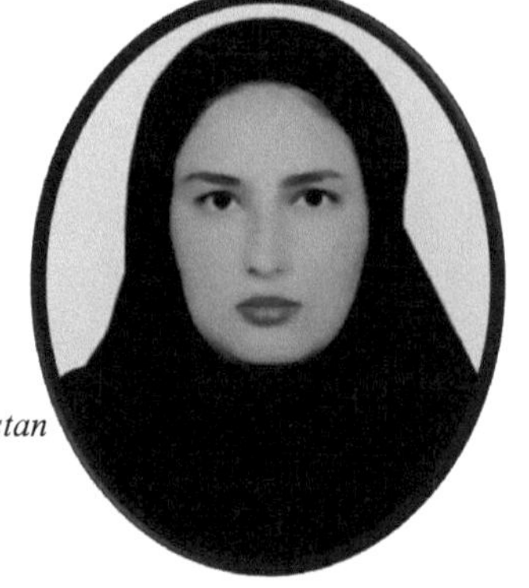

Ommolbanin Az

Nursing Expert, Third Rank in 2013, Graduated from Larestan University, Fars, Iran

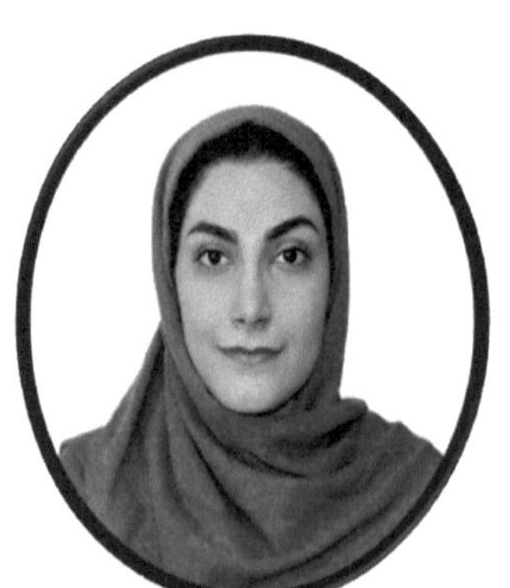

Forough Ameri

Anesthesiology Resident at Iran University of Medical Science, Tehran, Iran

This Book is dedicated to

My Family's

Content

Chapter I

Introduction

Introduction

The etiology of concussion varies from country to country, but the most important factor is vehicle accidents. 50% of the victims are vehicle occupants. Motorcyclists, pedestrians, cyclists, etc. are in the next stages. 150,000 deaths from head injuries occur annually in the United States. The third leading cause of death (after heart disease and cancer) in this country and also the first leading cause of death in people under 45 years and 78% of deaths in the age group of 15-24 years is brain trauma. In the United States, 500,000 head trauma patients are admitted to hospitals each year, of which 50,000 die before reaching hospital and 450,000 are admitted per year, 10% of whom have moderate head trauma and 10% Severe head injuries. Of the hospitalized patients, 15,000 to 20,000 die and 50,000 have permanent disabling complications. The number of brain injuries in the world is high, but in Iran due to the high number of road accidents, these injuries are more frequent, so that in 2007 more than 22918 people in the country died in road accidents. In Sweden, meanwhile, deaths from accidents are 150-200 per year.

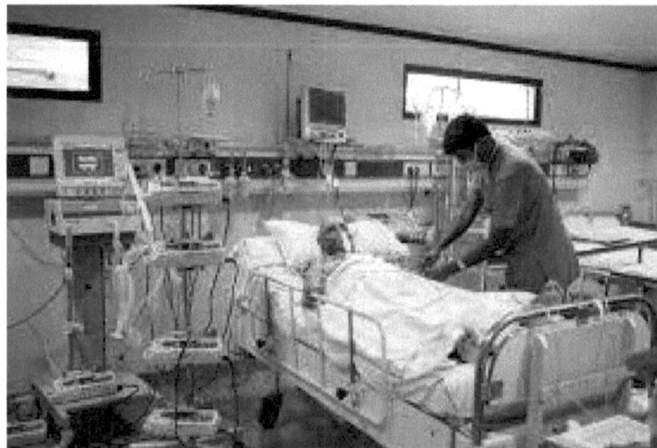

Figure 1. Government-funded critical care training to launch for nurses

On the other hand, recent advances in medical science and the improvement of care services have increased the number of survivors of these injuries, but these advances have not guaranteed a return to pre-injury health in them. Today, more than 7.3 million

Americans live with disabilities due to brain injuries. Findings from the study by Lippert Gruner et al. (2003) on 24 severe coma patients admitted to the ICU indicate that 6 patients died, 3 patients remained in vegetative state, 6 patients with severe disabilities and 6 patients with moderate disabilities. Were infected and only 3 patients recovered well after one year. Coma patients experience a variety of changes, including cognitive changes and physical disabilities, behavioral problems, and lack of sense and cognition, which have significant effects on the life of the patient and his family.

Most stroke patients are admitted to the intensive care unit, and these patients are in an environment of sensory deprivation, stress, and anxiety based on the cause of the injury. One of the dangers that threatens the patient in the ICU is sensory deprivation, which is caused by a decrease in the reception of sensory stimuli or sensory stimuli that are unregulated and meaningless, which can impair the healing process of nerve damage. Forgetfulness and damage to short-term memory.

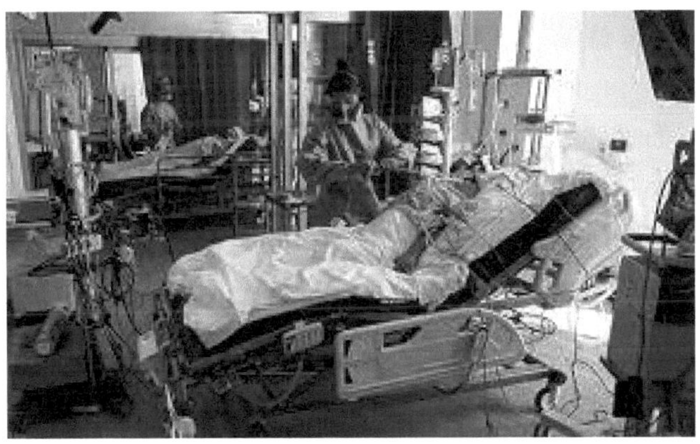

Figure 2. Why the ICU nursing shortage can be ignored no longer

Mental and cognitive function is the basis of people's interaction with the environment and is in fact the mental and psychological part of brain function. The first mental function, awakening and reacting to the environment, is called consciousness. One of the complications of sensory deprivation is abnormal mental function. Abnormal mental function is one of the most well-known symptoms of dangerous diseases. More than 80% of ICU patients develop mental disorders and these disorders increase the patient mortality 3 times and also increase the length of stay in the ICU and dependence on the ventilator. In the United States, 66% of patients who have been hospitalized in the ICU for at least 10 days have experienced complications of sensory deprivation during hospitalization and after discharge.

One of these complications is psychosis, 30 to 80% of cases of psychosis depend on comorbidities, prescribing various drugs and sensory deprivation. A study in Denmark found that 39% of patients admitted to the ICU developed psychosis. Complications of sensory deprivation can affect the level of consciousness. In Iran, there are no accurate statistics on sensory deprivation in ICU patients, but Aghazadeh et al. No sensory burden). But the study of emotional reactions showed that 39.8% experience pain, 18.5% anxiety, 12% fear, 7.4% violence and anger, and 9% hatred, which seems to be due to Sensory deprivation due to lack of family visits. Therefore, he suggested increasing the number of visits to patients in special wards.

For the first time in the 1950s, the Pennsylvania institute for human potential achievement advocated the idea that using coma stimulation programs by providing environmental inputs for all five senses at one frequency, intensity, and duration could improve coma and degree of recovery. Possibly improves synaptic nervousness. The results of Carter and Di Yang (1989) research also support the above idea.

In general, it can be concluded that one of the main and determining needs in the recovery process of ICU patients and preventing sensory deprivation and its complications such as delirium and impaired consciousness, is to perform appropriate and balanced sensory stimulation for patients.

Vision stimulation is performed using a flashlight at a time when the patient's eyes open spontaneously or there is a lash reflex or moving objects within the patient's field of vision. Hearing stimulation is possible even in a low-noise environment by explaining the activities and calling the patient by name and giving temporal or spatial information. Touch is one of the strongest and most basic senses. It also expresses emotions such as peace and security more effectively as a form of communication.

Nurses and family members can use touch in all aspects of patient care and observe patient response.

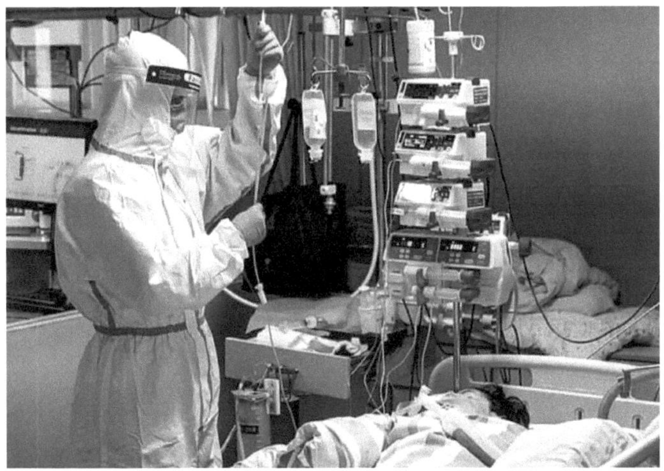

Figure 3. Honouring ICU Nurses as Healthcare Heroes

Motor stimulation is done to improve a person's perception or awareness of the surrounding space. Changing the patient's position from one position to another and the range of motion of the joints, as part of the stimulation program, helps prevent the effects of immobility.

Odor stimulation activates the nervous system and limbic system. In response to different odors, the patient may move his lips or nose or assume a sniffing state. Providing a regular program including sensory stimulation of vision, hearing, smell, touch, and movement is an effort to achieve maximum recovery for these patients; Because excessive or low stimuli cause behavioral changes in patients who have little understanding of their environment and each person needs a certain level of environmental stimulation to maintain and maintain life.

On the other hand, ICU patients' families, in addition to their role in patient care, also have a series of problems and needs, because the constant presence behind the door of a room where one of the most important family members is present, needs help and He is in such a critical condition that it is possible not to see him forever at any moment, it can impose great psychological pressure on the family.

The general health of the family may be endangered due to concerns about the patient's condition, feelings of inadequacy to save the patient, lack of confidence in the proper and adequate care of the patient by staff, this problem sometimes in the form of aggression, staff protests and complaints to superiors. Indicates. All of these factors can endanger the general health of the family. As in Khorramabad Nomadic Martyrs Hospital, many verbal and physical clashes are observed daily between the staff and the patient's companions.

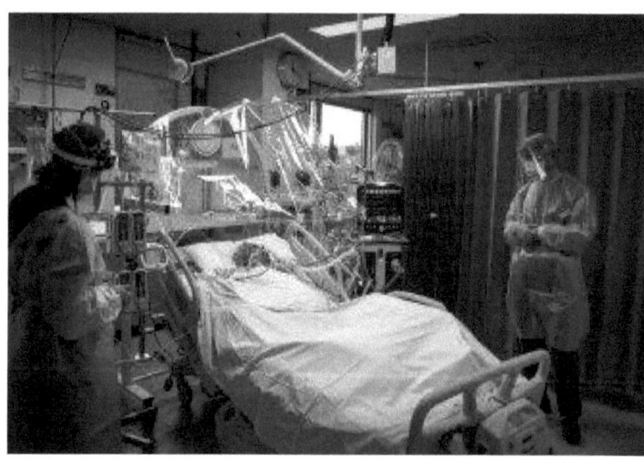

Figure 4. COVID's strain on health system also a drain on intensive care studies

The policy of family visitation of patients admitted to the intensive care unit currently has many limitations. However, family and family life are an essential part of every person's health, the family should be considered as important in the nursing intervention program as the patient himself in terms of the importance and role it plays for the patient.

Today, the care environment includes patients and families and general care includes family and patient care. For some reason, this continuity in family involvement is not always possible and the family moves away from the patient. One of these cases is hospitalization in the intensive care unit, which due to the philosophy and structure of such wards, the presence of family members is prohibited and visits are severely limited. At present, these restrictions apply to almost all teaching and private hospitals in Iran, but in any case, the issue of visiting patients, both humanely and in Islam, is a duty with a spiritual reward and a duty.

In addition, treatment decisions are complex and communication is necessary to design therapies in which the patient's values must be taken into account, and communication also affects the patient and family's treatment outcomes.

Therefore, ensuring high-level family relationships is a priority for nurses, physicians, professional communities and legal organizations. However, time constraints, lack of communication skills training, unclear goals, ambiguous processes, and other challenges affect family motivation and complicate communication. Current communications in the ICU are often inconsistent, inadequate and of poor quality.

Family members believe that if understandable and clear information reaches them every day, it can be very useful and effective. However, it is rare for families to receive sufficient and effective information. As a result, the patient's unique values and priorities may not be taken into account and costly treatments may make the dying process longer and more difficult for many patients.

Given the urgent need to improve communication with families, researchers have tested a variety of innovative approaches to this. For example, Leslie et al. (2010) conducted review studies using the latest domestic and foreign articles taken from reputable sites to examine the improvement of communication in the ICU and its impact on the patient, family and hospital costs.

The results of their study showed that in most of the experimental studies, the use of targeted print information, ethical consultations, conferences by ICU staff with the presence of patients' family members with the aim of familiarizing and informing about diagnostic and therapeutic methods, treatment goals, and full knowledge of the patient's values and assessment of family perception, reduce family anxiety, patient length of stay, and use of specific therapies, but conclusive evidence suggests that such interventions reduce the overall cost of treatment.

Currently, limited access is allowed in Tehran hospitals, and for the first time, a device for audio and video communication between patients and families has been installed in the CCU ward of Isa ibn Maryam Hospital in Isfahan. Hafez Hospital in Shiraz can have an online appointment with their patient.

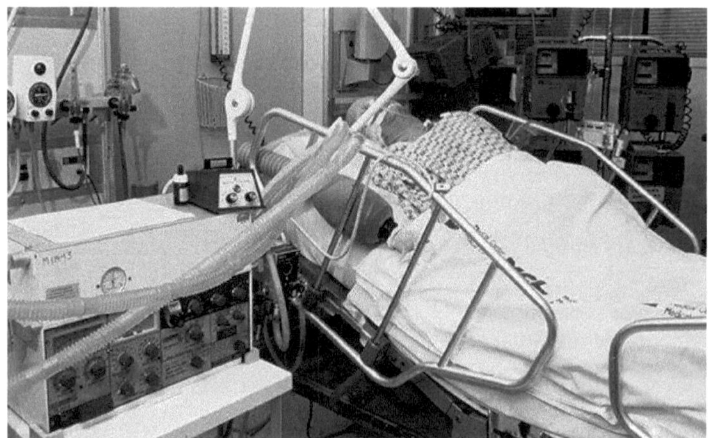

Figure 5. COVID-19: 'critical care nurse numbers can't keep pace with boost in supply of ICU beds'

In Khorramabad Social Security and Shahid Madani Hospitals, companions can see their patients through the window, but in Nomadic Martyrs Hospital, where most patients are from nomads and surrounding villages, there is a deeper emotional connection between the patient and the family.

The surgical and internal medicine ICU is on the second floor of the hospital, and there are no windows to see patients, and companions spend many hours behind the door waiting to hear from the patient. In addition, in most of the mentioned centers, sensory stimulation is performed by a nurse.

Also, in Iran, a study comparing the role of family and nurse in sensory stimulation has not been performed. Therefore, this study was designed and conducted to compare the effect of sensory stimulation by family members and nurses on the level of consciousness and vital signs of patients admitted to the ICU.

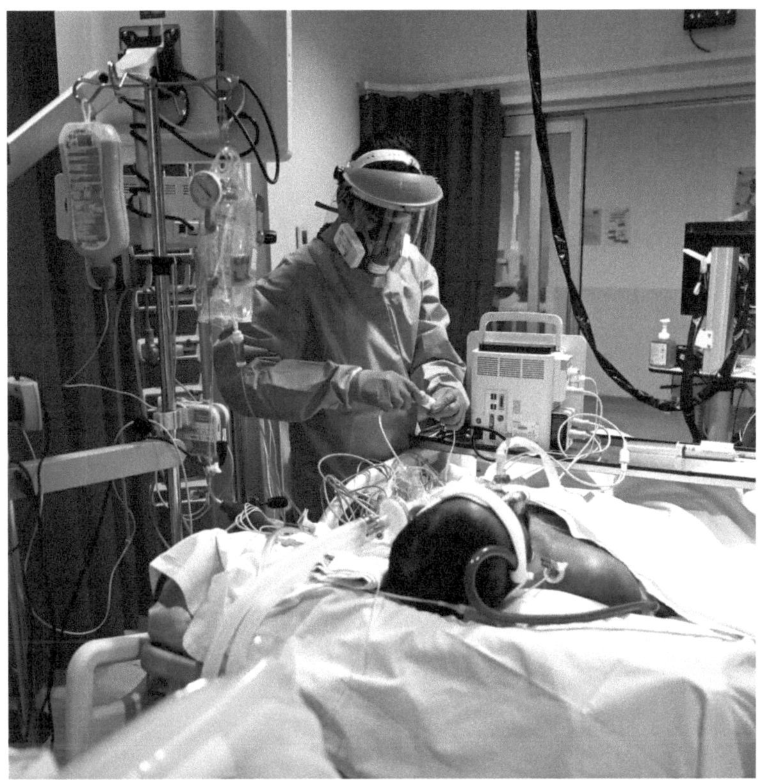

Figure 6. Critical care beds are no use without enough specialist staff

Chapter II

The Structure of the brain and its protective layers

The skull is a strong bone that surrounds the brain. The meninges prevent direct contact between the brain and the skull bone. These curtains from the inside to the inside consist of three layers called hard sham, spider and soft sham. It fills the cerebrospinal fluid between the arachnids and the soft palate (the space below the arachnids). There are 4 ventricles (cavities) in the brain in which cerebrospinal fluid also flows. The brain is made up of two hemispheres, the brain, the cerebellum and the brainstem.

The hemispheres of the brain are each divided into functional parts called lobes. These lobes include anterior lobe, temporal lobe, parietal lobe and occipital lobe. Each part of the brain has a specific function.

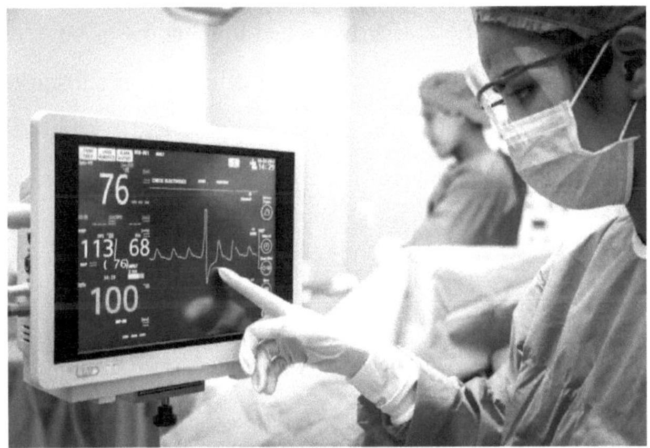

Figure 7. How to Become a Critical Care Nurse

Anterior lobe; Personality, problem solving, emotions, concentration, judgment, speech and voluntary movements, temporal lobe; Memory, hearing, taste, smell, language comprehension, organization, parietal lobe; Sense of touch, spatial perception, visual perception, differentiation of size, color and shapes from each other, occipital lobe; Vision, cerebellum; It controls balance, motor coordination, fine motor activity and brainstem, respiration, heart rate, level of consciousness, swallowing, sense of balance, and the sleep-wake cycle.

Brain blood circulation

The supply of oxygen and nutrients to the brain and neurons by the blood vessels provided by the circulatory system is called cerebral circulation. Oxygen consumption is relatively high in the brain and neurons, but their storage is very low.

Therefore, the number of blood vessels and capillaries in the brain tissue is very high, because it can meet the need for about 55 ml of blood per minute for every 100 grams of brain tissue. At rest, the adult brain accounts for about 15 percent of the heart's output. Only in cases such as decreased blood oxygen, increased carbon dioxide and hydrogen, increases the amount of blood supply to the brain. Increasing the concentration of hydrogen ions in the cerebral circulation weakens the activity of neurons. On the other hand, increasing hydrogen ions increases cerebral blood flow, which in turn removes both carbon dioxide and other acidic substances from brain tissues. The excretion of carbon dioxide reduces carbonic acid in brain tissue and, along with the release of other acids, reduces the concentration of hydrogen ions to normal levels.

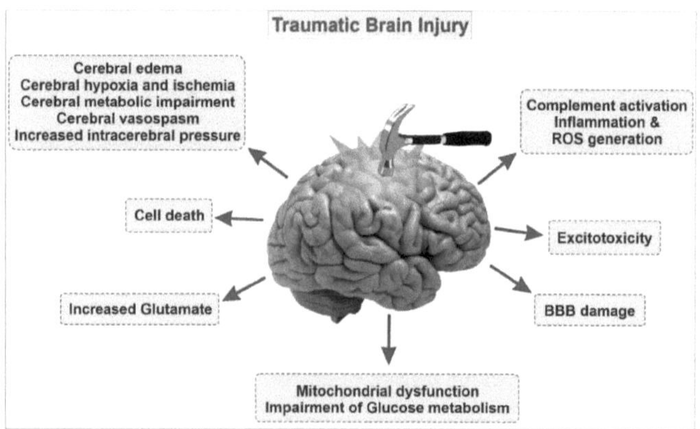

Figure 8. Traumatic Brain Injury and Blood–Brain Barrier (BBB)

Oxygen consumption in the brain is about 3.5 milliliters of oxygen per 100 grams of brain tissue per minute. When cerebral blood flow is insufficient and there is a lack of oxygen to the brain, a mechanism called vasodilation is activated, which increases blood flow and oxygen delivery to the brain tissues because the brain is located in the closed space of the skull. The amount of blood that reaches it should be considered so that it always remains constant and does not increase or decrease the pressure in the brain. More active areas of the brain are usually given more blood, so in right-handed people, the blood in the left hemisphere is slightly larger than in the right hemisphere. Also, in a person who is speaking, more blood is given to the forehead area on the left hemisphere, which is the center of speech, and in listeners, more blood is given to the temporal area, which is the hearing center in the brain.

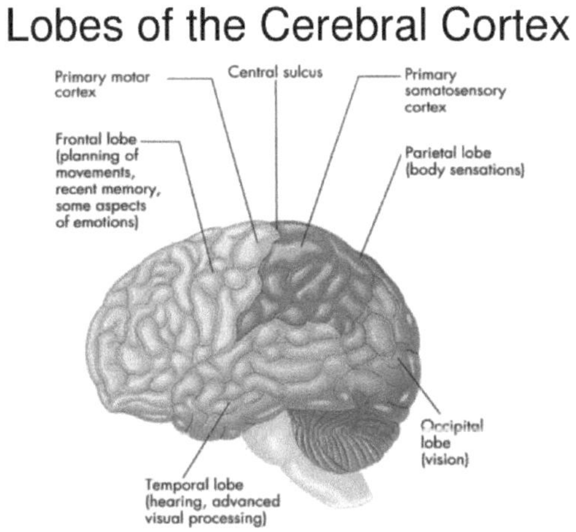

Figure 9. Cerebral cortex, Nervous system diagram, Somatosensory cortex

CSF

A clear, colorless fluid that is part of the blood plasma and circulates through the capillaries into the cerebral cavities. This fluid moves slowly between the nerve connective tissues and in addition to nourishing the tissue and disposing of waste products, it has a protective role in preventing the rupture of cerebral arteries when the body moves down and in cases where blood pressure rises in the cerebral arteries. This fluid passes through the meninges, ventricles, and subarachnoid space, then returns to the veins and finally to the bloodstream. This fluid acts as a lymph in other parts of the body. Increased volume of cerebrospinal fluid at an early age causes hydrocephalus and at an older age cause "brain swelling". The role of the sympathetic nervous system in regulating cerebral blood flow:

The circulatory system of the brain has a strong sympathetic nervous system that originates in the sympathetic terminals of the neck and ascends along the cerebral arteries. These nerves also innervate the smallest cerebral arteries inside the white matter. The most important role of the sympathetic nerves in regulating blood flow to the brain is to prevent stroke. Thus, when arterial blood pressure is greatly elevated in strenuous muscle activity, the sympathetic nerves narrow the large and medium-sized arteries sufficiently to prevent this high pressure from reaching the capillaries of the brain and causing them to rupture and bleed.

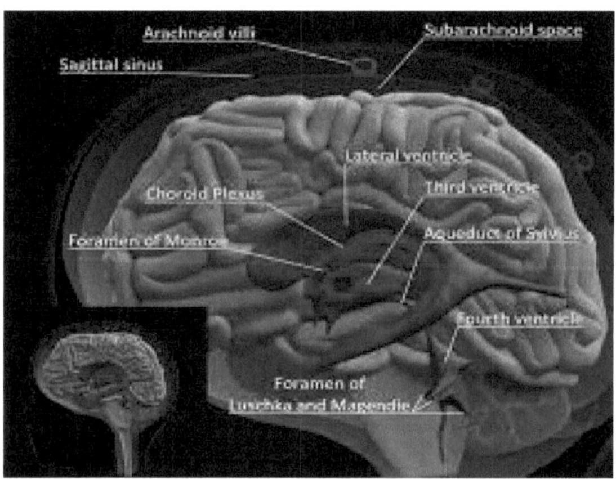

Figure 10. Cerebrospinal Fluid Dynamics Relevant to Hydrocephalus

Head injury

It is referred to as head trauma, which may include scalp injuries, skull fractures, and brain damage.

Types of head injuries based on the type of injury

Closed damage; In this case, the skull bone remains healthy. When the brain becomes swollen from trauma, because it is surrounded by the skull, the edema of the brain causes an increase in intracranial pressure. In this case, the brain tissue is compressed, which in turn leads to an increase in the size of the damage. Brain tissue may also penetrate into accessible cavities in the skull.

Like the eyeball, in which case by applying pressure to the optic nerves can cause dysfunction of the eye or dilation of the pupil. Open or penetrating damage; In this case, the object pierces the skull and penetrates hard into the palate or into the brain. Fractures and injuries to the skull may not be associated with brain damage, or in submerged skull fractures, a piece of broken bone may sink into the brain and damage the brain. Symptoms of concussion and dysfunction vary depending on the location of the trauma.

When the brain is damaged, a person's thinking, personality, and physical functions change. These changes may be transient or permanent. Damage to the functional lobes of the right and left brain can have different consequences. For example, damage to the right hemisphere of the brain reduces control over left-hand movements, and vice versa. In diffuse brain damage, both the left and right sides of the brain are involved. The consequences of brain damage are unpredictable. Brain damage can have a lasting effect on a patient's identity, personality, way of thinking, acting, and feeling. A concussion can change a patient's life in a matter of seconds. No two brain injuries are exactly alike. The effects of brain injury are complex and vary depending on factors such as the cause, location and severity of the injury.

Classification of brain injuries by location of impact

Traumatic brain injuries include focused and diffuse injuries.

Disseminated brain injuries

Diffuse brain injuries include concussion, diffuse axonal injury, and shaken infant syndrome. Concussion occurs in response to a sudden movement of the head (causing the brain to strike the bowl of the head), a direct blow to the head, a bullet, and a rapid shaking of the head.

Concussion is the most common type of brain injury, which can lead to blood vessels in the brain being damaged and the nerves in the brain damaged. Concussion may be asymptomatic without cranial fractures, bleeding, or edema. Symptoms include nausea and vomiting, dizziness, blurred vision, blurred vision, headache, forgetting events before or after a concussion (transient and less than 10 minutes), temporary loss of consciousness (less than 10 minutes). The person may not be anesthetized and may only feel dizzy), loss of balance, difficulty concentrating. Symptoms usually disappear after 72 hours. But the symptoms may last for months. Treatment for concussion involves complete rest under the supervision of a physician.

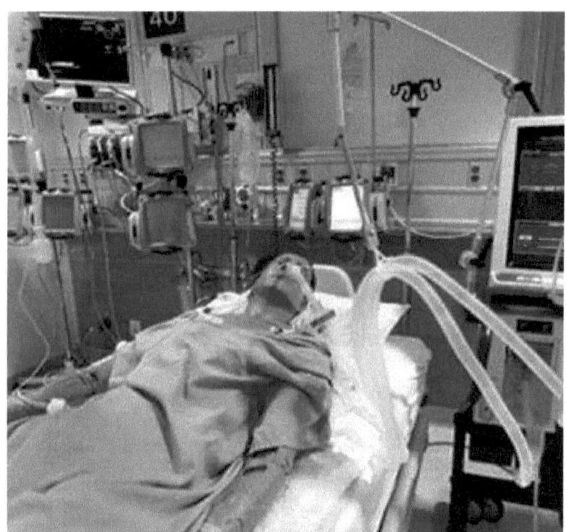

Figure 11. Global Critical Care Equipment Industry 2019, Deep Market Research Report, Analysis

A very important point about concussion is that activities that may lead to re-injury should be avoided until the symptoms of trauma are completely healed, because if the injuries from the first trauma are not completely healed. However, a blow to the head, even a not so strong blow, can lead to serious injury and even death. People who have symptoms of concussion for 15 minutes should stay out for a week, and people who lose consciousness following a concussion should have at least one month of activities that lead to injury.

Diffuse axonal damage is caused by severe shaking or severe head rotation. When the head shakes suddenly (in a whip) without hitting an object, a sudden increase or decrease in speed can damage the brain. Rupture of nerve tissue following this injury can disrupt the normal functioning of the brain and lead to general brain damage, coma and even death. Severe shaking of infants causes stretching and damage to delicate nerve cells and can lead to seizures, coma, permanent disability, and death. Rupture of blood vessels in the brain and cerebral hemorrhage cause accumulation of blood, which in turn causes compression of brain tissue and edema, which leads to brain damage.

Concentrated brain injuries

Concentrated brain injuries include brain crushing, brain edema, hematoma, and fluid accumulation in the brain. Brain crush refers to contusion and crushing of the cerebral cortex. When the head hits a solid object and vice versa. Cerebral edema increases intracranial pressure, which prevents blood from entering the scalp (to deliver glucose and oxygen to the brain). Increased intracranial pressure should be relieved by surgery or drainage of cerebrospinal fluid.

Hematoma refers to the accumulation of blood and blood clots due to rupture of blood vessels. And hydrocephalus refers to the accumulation of fluid in or around the brain. The brain has four ventricles in which cerebrospinal fluid flows. When blood enters these ventricles, the site of absorption of cerebrospinal fluid is blocked and cerebrospinal fluid accumulates in the brain. This accumulation increases pressure and damage to the brain.

Effects of head injury on level of consciousness

Generally, 8 abnormal states of consciousness include confusion, psychosis, astonishment, coma, vegetative state, stable vegetative state, minimal state of consciousness, syndrome, and brain death following a concussion.

Confused; It includes lack of awareness of time and place, lack of proper response to environmental stimuli, short and irrelevant responses; The patient wakes up with acoustic stimuli but is drowsy and falls asleep quickly. In the state of psychosis or delirium, in addition to the symptoms of meningitis, the patient has sweating, tachycardia (increased heart rate), trembling hands, forgetfulness, emotional and personality changes, discrete speech, disorganized thinking, hallucinations, rapid changes in mental states. (From lethargy to restlessness and vice versa), sometimes seizures and decreased sleep. In shock or stupor, the casualty is immobile and does not respond to normal stimuli, but can be briefly stimulated by strong stimuli such as painful stimuli (casualty screams or screams).

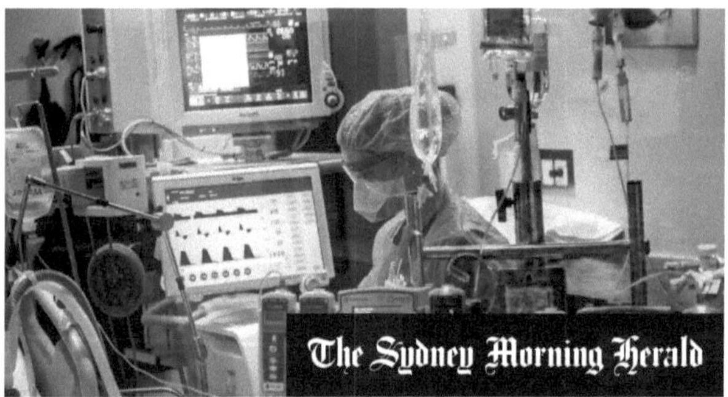

Figure 12. Australian COVID pandemic triggers mass exodus of critical care nurses

In a state of bewilderment, the person has little awareness of his or her surroundings. In the syndrome, the patient is alert and awake, but due to complete paralysis of the body (voluntary muscles) is unable to move the body and communicate with others. In this case, the person can only communicate with others by moving the eyes vertically or blinking. This condition is caused by damage to the lower parts of the brain (brainstem) and keeping the upper parts of the brain healthy. This condition usually has no cure.

Coma; A Greek word meaning deep sleep. Coma refers to a state of deep and stable anesthesia. The comatose patient cannot be awakened (even with painful physical stimuli), the patient does not respond to stimuli of light and pain, has no sleep-wake cycle, and is not aware of intentional and purposeful activities. The outcome of a coma depends on the cause, location, severity, and extent of the neurological damage, which varies from recovery to recovery to death. If the patient comes out of a coma, the recovery process is gradual, so that the patient wakes up for only a few minutes in the first days, this period of awakening gradually increases. People who come out of a coma experience a wide range of temporary and permanent physical, behavioral, mental, and psychological disorders. Coma rarely lasts more than 2-3 weeks. But it can last for months and years.

After a coma, either the patient enters a vegetative state (life) or dies. It is recommended in various sources that in addition to the patient who is in a coma or vegetative life, one should be careful in conversations because the patient may hear the words of others. Therefore, negative and frustrating conversations should be avoided. In the vegetative state, the patient is not conscious and unaware of his surroundings, lacks cognitive functions, but has a sleep-wake cycle and appears to be awake for short periods of time. It is also normal for breathing and digestion.

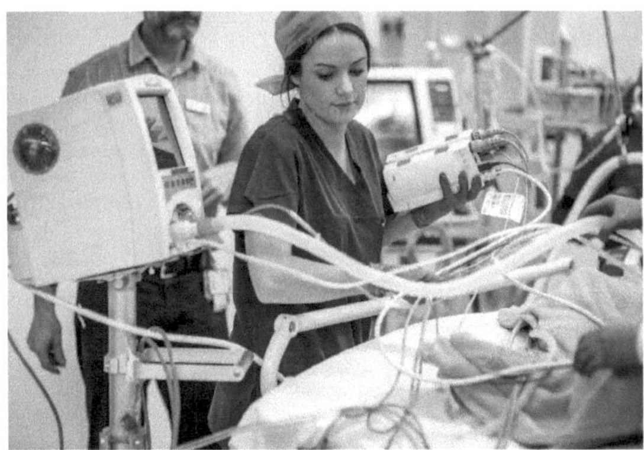

Figure 13. ICU Nurse Resume (Examples, Tips, Cover Letter)

In this case, the patient may open his eyes, make noise, or move. Unlike in a coma, the patient has his eyes open (usually in a fixed position or can follow objects). The patient may experience a sleep-wake cycle or a stable awakening. There is a general response to pain in the patient (increased heart rate and respiration rate). When this condition lasts for more than a month, it is called "stable vegetable condition".

The patient may have behaviors that indicate alertness, such as; Gritting teeth, swallowing, smiling, shedding tears, moaning and screaming occur without external stimuli. People who enter the vegetative stage may remain in this state for years. The younger the patient, the better his chances of recovery and full consciousness. Children have a 60 percent chance and adults have a 50 percent chance of recovering within 6 months, but after a year the chances of recovery are greatly reduced. Even if the patient regains consciousness after one year, he or she will usually suffer from major physical and mental disabilities for the rest of his or her life.

In the conscious state, the patient seems to be at least in a state of vegetative life, but is able to process information, develop initial reflexes, follow simple commands, and be aware of environmental stimuli, but brain death to a complete cessation. Refers to brain activity, which is irreversible. In this case, the patient is able to continue his plant life only with the help of ventilator and the patient will die as soon as the device is removed. So, in fact, it is a state of deep unconsciousness or non-response to environmental stimuli caused by traumatic injuries (accidents, falls, fights and sports accidents) or non-traumatic brain injuries (infections, epilepsy, metabolic causes, cerebrovascular diseases) Traumatic cranial trauma, malignancies, and central nervous system surgeries occur, and the GCS is a measure of the severity and degree of coma. The main components of this scale include eye opening and response, verbal response and motor response.

Diagnostic methods in head trauma patients

Various methods are used to evaluate patients with head trauma, especially when entering the emergency room. These methods include clinical and paraclinical trials. Among these, the most important method of assessing the type, extent and progression of head injury is to perform CTs of the brain. CTs are one of the most effective tools used in neurological emergencies, both traumatic and non-traumatic conditions. X-rays are absorbed to different degrees in different tissues. Higher, denser structures, such as bone, absorb more radiation, and vice versa, parts such as air and fat do not absorb radiation at all. To interpret any graph from any part of the body, one must first know the main structure of that part. Skull CTs are no exception to this rule in order to identify pathological cases. Success in interpreting head CTs depends on familiarity with different structures from cortical tissue to the vascular system, ventricles, and ducts. Knowing the neural function of different areas of the brain helps to interpret the findings during a physical examination.

As cardiologists use fixed methods to read ECGs such as rhythm, rhythm, heart axis, it is better to use such methods in the interpretation of CTs to prevent misdiagnosis [46]. When interpreting CTs, all states must be kept in mind, because the presence of one pathological condition cannot rule out the rest. Acute bleeding in CTs is seen as hyperdense and light in color, and this is because the globin molecule absorbs X-rays. As the bleeding progresses and the globin molecule is destroyed, the state of hyperdense will disappear. In CTs, the density of the blood approaches the density of the brain within 4 to 2 weeks.

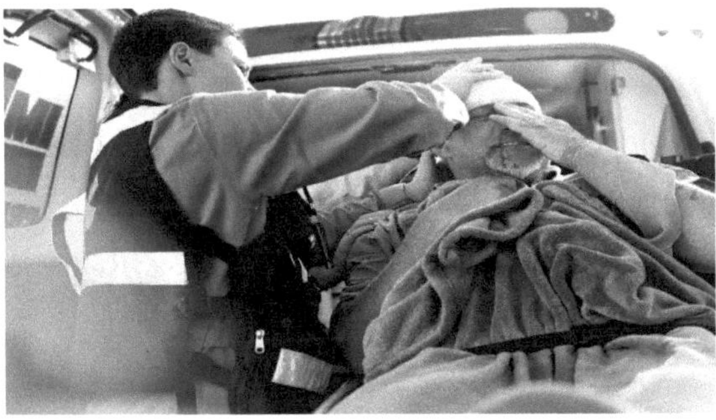

Figure 14. Frontal Lobe Head Trauma Effects and Treatment

Of course, this time also depends on the amount of bleeding and eventually darkens than the brain itself (during 2-3 weeks). Epidural hemorrhage is most often seen in the form of a lens above the cerebral cortex. The main cause of this type of bleeding in 85% of cases is meningeal artery rupture. It is less likely to cause this type of venous bleeding. If treatment is started immediately, the probability of death is less than 20%. Subdural hemorrhage is a sickle or crescent hemorrhage that can occur between the brain or the tantrum. This bleeding is seen in the area between the sutures or slits and can be seen as an acute or delayed complication that in both cases can be due to rupture of superficial or communication vessels. Acute subdural hemorrhage is more commonly seen following compression injuries and is often associated with severe brain injury that has a poor prognosis. Which causes the death of 60-80% of patients with severe injuries. Delayed subdural hemorrhage occurs because in intracranial injuries, a clot may stop the bleeding and put the patient at risk for bleeding in subsequent injuries.

The picture of bleeding on CTs depends on when the bleeding started. In subdural hemorrhage that is not detectable, contrast injection can be used. CTs can also be reliable for small hematomas as small as 5 mm. non-traumatic blood pressure-related injuries are more common in the elderly and at the site of the underlying complications. Bleeding for these reasons can cause blood to enter the ventricular space, which is seen in CTs with bleeding in the ventricular space.

Traumatic intracerebral hemorrhage may be visible immediately after injury. Intraventricular hemorrhage can be due to causes such as; Trauma, high blood pressure with a ruptured ventricle or subarachnoid hemorrhage can occur with a ruptured ventricle. About 10% of this type of bleeding is due to trauma. Hydrocephalus can occur regardless of the cause. Subarachnoid hemorrhage is mostly due to trauma, tumors, arteriovenous abnormalities and severe vertebral malformations, but in 10-15% of cases the cause is unknown and hydrocephalus is the cause of 20% of subarachnoid hemorrhage.

The ability of CTs to detect this type of bleeding depends on several factors, such as; Scanner type, bleeding time, skill in interpreting CTs. In 98-95% of cases, this type of bleeding is detected in CTs in the first 1-12 hours after the attack. The appearance of the brain on CTs is white and gray, a combination that is clearly seen in adults and is quite symmetrical. For example, in stroke, this division of white and gray disappears, and in metabolic disorders, this disorder is seen in the border of white and gray. Abscesses are also seen as a low-density area or hypotenuse in CTs without contrast. Strokes are either hemorrhagic or non-hemorrhagic. Non-hemorrhagic strokes can be seen in the first 2-3 hours of an attack, but in most cases it takes about 12-24 hours to be seen on CTs.

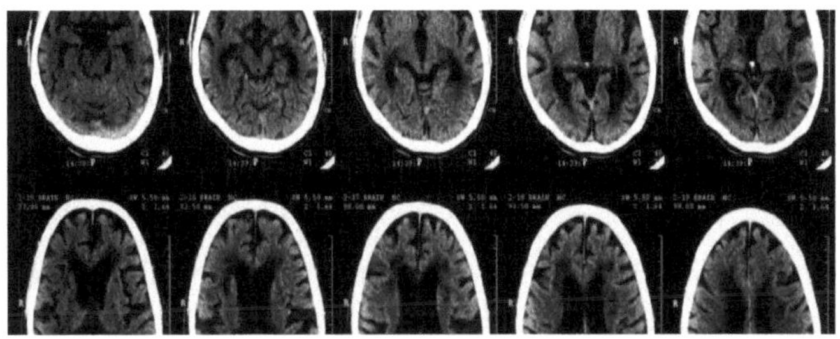

Figure 15. How do healthcare providers diagnose traumatic brain injury (TBI)?

The fastest change seen in the ischemic area is the disappearance of the distinction between white and gray area, which can be a very important and accurate finding at first. Edema can be seen in approximately 70% of attacks and is usually seen between 3-5 days at the latest. Small lacunar strokes follow high blood pressure and are seen in the basal ganglia.

Diagnosing a skull fracture can be a bit difficult due to the presence of wrinkles on the skull structure. Fractures can occur anywhere on the skull. Fractures are divided into compressive and non-compressive. A fracture in the skull bone can also indicate damage to the inside of the brain. The presence of air inside the skull can indicate that the skull and sternum are damaged. Basilar fractures are more common in the hard part. The maxillary, ethmoid, and sphenoid 3 sinuses should be perfectly clear and visible, but if there is fluid in these sinuses, it indicates a fracture and damage to the skull.

In general, most trauma patients are admitted to the intensive care unit, and these patients are in an environment of sensory deprivation, stress, and anxiety, which is unregulated and meaningless due to reduced sensory or sensory stimuli. Sensory deprivation can disrupt the healing process of a nerve lesion. For this reason, here we will discuss sensory deprivation in the ICU, its complications, and the role of sensory stimulation.

Sensory deprivation in the ICU and the role of sensory stimulation

As mentioned in the statement, the patient with a concussion is placed in a sensory deprivation environment based on the type of injury. In fact, the patient who is admitted to the intensive care unit on the one hand due to critical conditions and damage to the structures responsible for maintaining wakefulness and alertness, prolonged immobility, isolation from the community and special conditions of special wards and on the other hand he is subject to sensory deprivation due to the complex treatment procedures that are performed on him; One of the main reasons for this can be the environment and unfamiliar people.

Most patients admitted to intensive care units, especially ICUs, do not visit their families until the end of the hospitalization period. Unfortunately, due to the high mortality rate in these departments, the patient may never be able to see his family in this world. Severe patients experience more or less stress while under intensive care, and anxiety is seen in most patients admitted to the intensive care unit. Exposure to various stressors such as illness, lack or anticipation of absence, hospitalization that are stressful factors can cause anxiety in the patient and anxiety is one of the preconditions of sensory deprivation.

Therefore, not paying attention to the client's psychological and social infrastructure and his privacy and perception will cause a feeling of invasion of the territory and the occurrence of emotional reactions and emotional deprivation, and the client's irritability and conditions such as violence and anger. Facilitates mental suffering and anxiety and delusions, all of which are manifestations of sensory deprivation. According to these findings, sensory deprivation of ICU patients and its complications should be avoided. Psychologists and teachers have long recognized the importance of sensory perceptions, but their importance in health and nursing has become apparent in the last two or three decades. Researchers believe that if a person is deprived of stimuli or receives excessive stimulation, his physical or mental balance is lost and behavioral changes such as auditory hallucinations, vision, anxiety and anxiety occur in him.

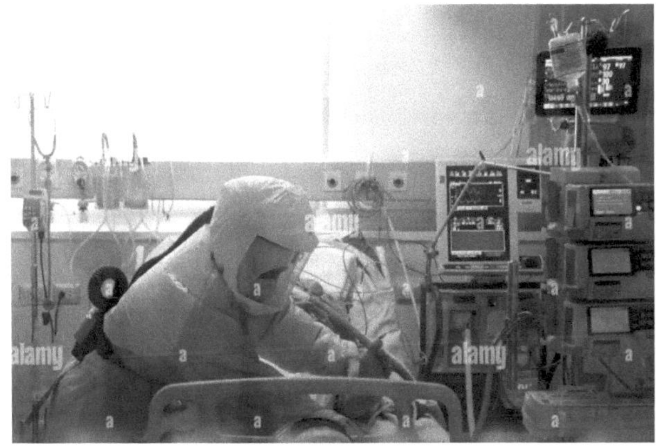

Figure 16. ICU Nurse High Resolution Stock Photography and Images

On the other hand, rehabilitation in ICU patients is a complex and long process that starts from the intensive care unit and continues in the community context. Proper and early rehabilitation helps to improve brain function and, of course, the individual's return to society. Rehabilitation has reached an acceptable standard for sensory, motor, behavioral, and cognitive problems, but there is controversy about consciousness disorder. Sensory stimulation interventions can be one of the rehabilitation methods that can be done in the hope of increasing the activity of the retina system and increasing awakening. In addition, despite the fact that brain damage is a process that lasts for hours and weeks, but the brain has the ability to permanently repair and repair and is activated immediately after the injury and modulates the organization and function of the brain. Coma stimulation awakens the brain by awakening the retinal activation system, or in lateral healthy nerve fibers under the influence of stimuli, lateral relationships are created that help reorganize brain activity.

In the past, the neurophysiological view of compensating for the lack of functions created by injury has been the organization of neural pathways. It has also been emphasized in these patients that treatment increases the use of different or less commonly used neuronal circuits. This condition is known as neurophysiological functional change in the central nervous system. Studies have shown that whenever a damaged system comes into operation, the rate of recovery is greater and faster. These studies show that sensory stimuli accelerate the growth of dendrites. It is hypothesized that the growth of dendrites is involved in the development of intelligence and adaptive behavior in humans.

In general, the nervous system functions as a sensory-motor feedback system through integration. If we deprive this system of intra-sensory institutions, human behaviors will become disorganized. Sensory deprivation impairs synaptic development and growth and delays the myelination of fibers, and an environment rich in stimuli has the opposite effect. The neurophysiological structural basis of plasticity seems to be based on synaptic changes that occur through hypertrophy and the germination of additional synapses. Therefore, it can be said that the ability of neurons to adapt or improve depends on factors such as; Activation of inactive neurons, which may have been previously inactive, is the ability of neurons adjacent to the lesion site to produce lateral axons that produce new synapses and changes in transmitter sensitivity. Depends on the chemicals.

Accordingly, as well as the use of sensory inputs in sensory-motor methods, to compensate for any nerve damage, the nervous system must be pressurized through sensory bombardment. Since coma patients are dependent on the nurse in all aspects of care and in the ICU wards all care of these patients is done by nurses, the nurse should identify the appropriate types of sensory stimuli with the help of the patient's family and present them according to different programs. Sensory stimuli provide an environment rich in meaningful stimuli for the patient. In the meantime, the use of familiar sensory stimuli has been emphasized.

The role and family needs of ICU patients

Hospitalization in special wards is a crisis for the patient and the family and causes great stress and anxiety for them. Nurses also show different behaviors in dealing with the phenomenon of family visits of patients admitted to the intensive care unit, which can be due to various problems for the hospitalized patient and also problems in the administration of the ward.

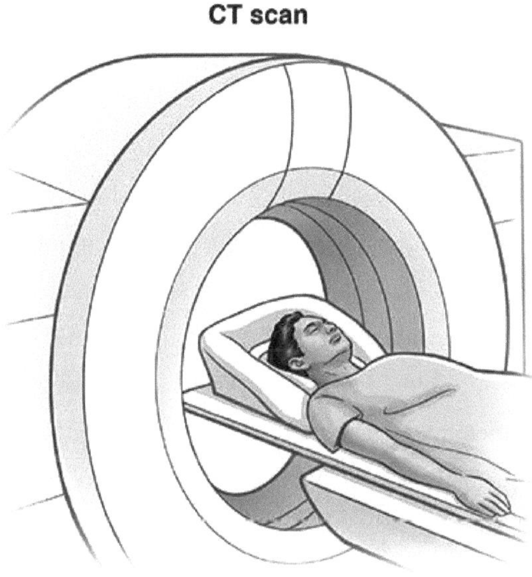

Figure 17. Head Injury

However, the existence of such a belief about close family visits with the patient can affect the quality of nursing care, especially its spiritual and spiritual dimensions. Alfred Adler believes that the basic problem in human beings is the feeling of inferiority and all the activities of the individual are done with the intention of becoming powerful, thus the activities of each individual is a kind of compensation to eliminate the feeling of inferiority and gain a more important sense. This can be a clear example for family members who are behind the ICU, as the factors that contribute to mental health disorders and treatment include biological factors, emotional and psychological factors, and social factors. The concept of public health is in fact an aspect of the general concept of health and refers to all methods and measures that are used to prevent mental illness and stress is an important response in people's lives, and even their ability to adapt to new situations, are good or bad. There are differing views on stress, including the definition of stress as a factor that increases the level of corticosteroid hormones and calls it a threat to the homeostasis of organisms that can react show emotional.

Examining critically ill patients and their families is an essential skill for intensive care staff. Today, the concept of family is not a simple concept and is defined beyond the meaning of love and support, regardless of legal and social boundaries. Families may have a positive effect on the patient's ability to adapt and recover from severe illness. Each family system is unique and varies in values, culture, religion, pre-crisis experiences, social and economic status, mental health, role expectations, communication patterns, health beliefs, and age. Assessing the needs and resources of the family is important to provide interventions that have the greatest impact on the patient and increase their interaction with the treatment team. There is strong evidence for the effect of family existence on the recovery of intensive care unit patients.

Family members can help the patient adapt to the environment and reduce anxiety and be a source of support for the patient. Creating a trusting relationship and working with the family is in everyone's best interest and can lead to the best performance. Studies show that there are many differences between the nurse and family views on family needs priorities.

Therefore, it is very important that the views and needs of the family are directly expressed and nursing interventions are designed based on these needs. Family members need to make sure that the best care is provided to the patient. This creates a sense of security in the family and a more realistic perspective. Family members need to always have access to their loved ones. With this in mind, it is important to reform a number of policies in meeting the sector. The number of people visiting at a time, age restrictions, times not visited and how to access the ward are some of the issues that need to be discussed. There is growing evidence that supports the presence of family members during surgical procedures and during cardiopulmonary resuscitation. Although this is controversial, family members feel comfortable and grateful to be with their loved ones.

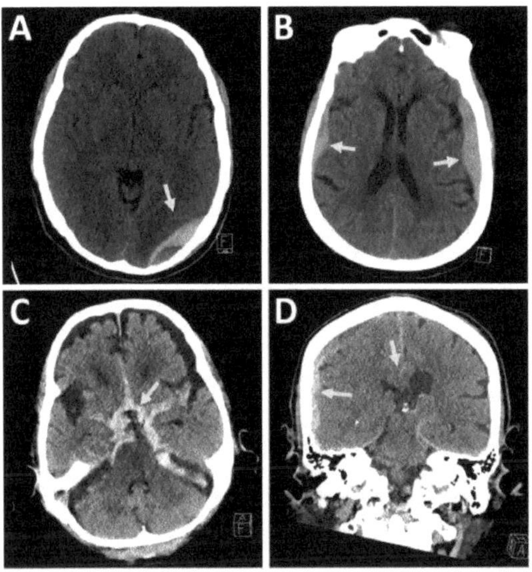

Figure 18. Neuroimaging of Traumatic Brain Injury

In the field of sensory deprivation in the ICU, its causes, how to deal with it and how to support the family of ICU patients, various studies have been conducted in the country and abroad, which are mentioned here.

In 2006, Aghazadeh et al. conducted a descriptive study on the sensory experiences of patients admitted to special wards of one of Ardabil hospitals with the aim of further familiarizing nurses with patients' sensory experiences and adjusting sensory stressors. Questionnaire and descriptive statistics were used to analyze the information. The questionnaire consisted of three parts; The first part includes demographic characteristics and clinical condition of the patient, the second part includes 40 closed-ended questions to determine olfactory, perceptual, visual, auditory, tactile and range of sensory perceptions, and the last part includes 6 open-ended questions to assess patients' emotional reactions from Such as anxiety, fear, sadness, pain, anger, peace and hatred and sin. The results of the above research showed that in more than 80% of the cases, the studied units experienced no unpleasant sensation at all, or only in some cases (no sensory overload). But the study of emotional reactions showed that 39.8% had experienced pain, 18.5% anxiety, 12% fear, 7.4% violence and anger, and 9% hatred, which seems to be due to deprivation. Feeling we have 'Run out of gas' emotionally. Therefore, he suggested increasing the number of visits to patients in special wards.

Regarding the effect of sensory stimulation on the level of consciousness of patients, Basampour et al. In a quasi-experimental study aimed at investigating the effect of organized auditory stimulation on the level of consciousness of coma patients in 2007 Available and random sampling with simultaneous group matching were performed in both intervention and control groups. Patients in the intervention group received hearing stimulation twice a day for 6 weeks, 6 days a week, at least 30 minutes apart with a tape recorder (5 to 15 minutes) from the voice of their loved one in the family, and the control group received only routine care. The level of consciousness of the patients in the intervention group was assessed before and after each stimulation session (4 times a day). The level of consciousness of patients in the control group was assessed 4 times a day with similar time intervals. The results showed that the mean level of consciousness of patients on the first day before the intervention and the fourteenth day after the intervention was statistically significant, while in the control group there was no significant difference.

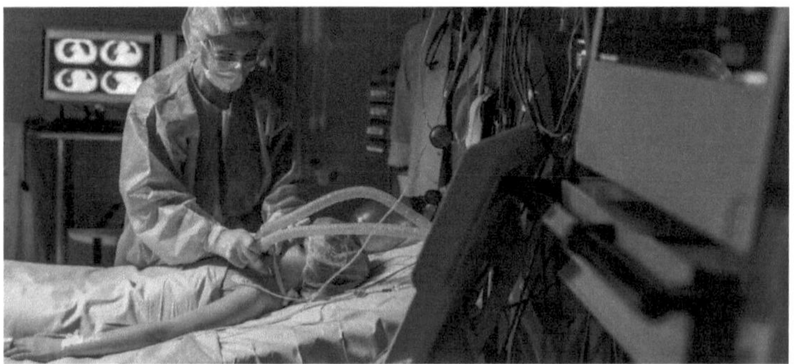

Figure 19. Learn About Teaching in Your Fast-Paced ICU

On the other hand, despite the similarity of the mean level of consciousness of patients in both groups on the first day before the intervention, there was a statistically significant difference between the mean level of consciousness of the two groups on the fourteenth day after the intervention. Therefore, the results of the above study showed that auditory stimulation with a familiar voice had a positive effect on improving the level of consciousness of coma patients. Provide ICU wards.

Also, a quasi-experimental study was conducted in 2008 by Shadfar et al. To investigate the effect of sensory stimuli on changes in the level of consciousness of comatose patients caused by concussions. For this study, 76 comatose patients due to concussion who were hospitalized in the intensive care unit of Shahid Kamyab Relief Hospital in Mashhad were selected. Patients were identified and a sensory stimulation program was performed for 12 hours for 2 weeks. In order to collect information, sample selection form, demographic information form, Glasgow coma table and Di Yang (1987) and Hilton (1994) sensory stimulation program were used. The results of the above study showed that during the hospitalization of coma patients in both experimental and control groups who used sensory stimulation in the first week and a total of two weeks, a significant difference was observed. The statistical test confirmed the researcher's hypothesis that the length of hospital stays of concussion patients who used sensory stimuli was shorter. At the end of the study, the researchers suggested that in future research, the effect of sensory stimulation by the patient's family on the level of consciousness and length of hospital stay in coma patients should be investigated.

Kavousipour et al. (2007) in an experimental and interventional study with the aim of comparing the increase in level of consciousness following sensory stimulation in both early and late times and through repeated measures, 21 men whose GCS in 3 days after trauma 8 or lower was randomly assigned to 3 groups of comparison, early intervention and late intervention. All patients were followed up until day 25 after trauma and their level of consciousness was assessed by GCS and CRS-R criteria every other day. One-week sensory stimulation intervention was presented by stimulating 5 senses of hearing, sight, touch, movement and smell in the early group from day 5-7 after trauma and in the late group from day 15 after trauma.

Also, during the week of the intervention, the patient's level of consciousness was assessed daily before and after receiving the intervention. Data were analyzed using paired t-test, Pearson correlation and repeated measures. The results of the above study showed that the analysis of the trend of changes in the level of consciousness during the first 25 days after trauma indicates a significant increase in the score of the two criteria in all three groups (P <0.001). Comparison of GCS score changes in 3 groups by post hoc post hoc test did not show a significant difference between the 3 groups (P = 0.15), but CRS-R score variations in early and late groups showed a significant difference (P=0.05).

Therefore, awakening of coma patients during spontaneous 25 days after trauma in all 3 groups. The findings of this study also indicated that the provision of sensory stimulation can accelerate this process of spontaneous healing.

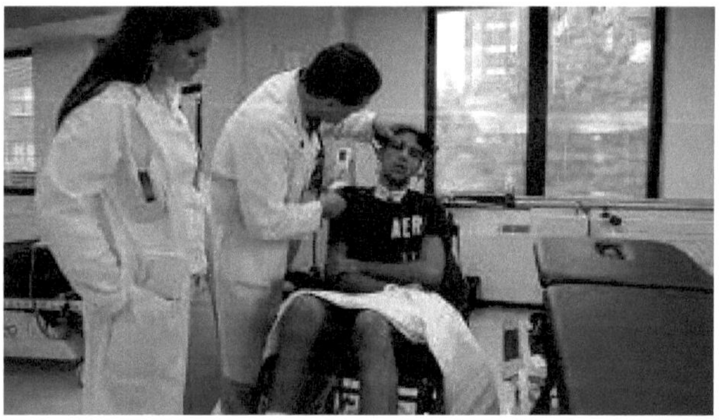

Figure 20. Overview of Traumatic Brain Injury

Regarding the effect of visits and sensory stimuli on patients' vital signs, Ashrafpour et al. The sample of this study consisted of 60 patients. Samples were selected randomly. Data collection tools in the above study were the form of recording hemodynamic measurements of arterial blood pressure, heart rate per minute and heart rate of patients and the necessary information was collected through a blood pressure monitor by a mercury sphygmomanometer and electrocardiogram recording. Blood pressure measurement and electrocardiogram recording were performed for all units in four stages, 5 minutes before the appointment and 5 minutes after the appointment, 5 minutes after the appointment and half an hour after the appointment. To monitor the patients' heart rhythm and determine the heart rate per minute, the electrocardiogram of the derivation II was recorded in each stage for 30 seconds by a central monitor. The number of visitors and the duration of the meeting were the same for all research units. Thus, the number of visitors was 2 and the duration of the meeting was 10 minutes. The research data were analyzed using descriptive and inferential statistics. T-test was used to compare the changes in heart rate and systolic and diastolic blood pressure and the relationship between these changes and demographic factors and disease-related characteristics.

The findings of the above study in relation to the objectives of the study showed that the number of systolic and diastolic blood pressure heart rate of the study units increases after the appointment compared to before the appointment and the increase of these parameters continues throughout the visit.

However, after the end of the visit, their amount decreased so that in the half an hour after the visit, the number of cytolic and diastolic blood pressure heart beats was less than in the pre-visit stage. Other findings of the above study showed that only the number of premature ventricular contractions increased during the visit but the visit had no effect on other heart disorders.

Kamranifar et al. Also conducted a study with the aim of determining the physiological parameters of patients before, during and after visits to CCU wards in Imam Khomeini Hospital in Ardabil in 2009. This was a descriptive evaluation study in which 50 patients with acute myocardial infarction were studied by available sampling method. The research tool included a questionnaire and a cardiac monitoring device. Use and reliability were obtained by calibration of the device.

For statistical analysis, analysis of variance with repeated measures was used. Findings The above study showed that changes in systolic, diastolic and mean arterial blood pressure, heart rate, respiration rate, temperature and percentage of arterial blood oxygen saturation before, during and after the visit were statistically significant (P <0.001), in such a way that the mentioned indicators have increased after the beginning of the meeting and there is a statistically significant difference with the time before the meeting (P <0.05) and Lee after at the end of the meeting, these indicators decreased again and there was no statistically significant difference with its value before the meeting (P> 0.05).

Regarding family visits with ICU patients, the findings of Marie Bezhap et al. (2007) with the aim of designing and describing a care plan in relation to family presence, to separate patients from the ventilator, showed that 46% of family members who They are present during the separation of the patient from the device, they have played a role in the proper care of the patient and easier and more effective separation by touching and talking to the patient.

Of course, there were some cases that had the opposite result, but in general, the results of the above research showed that the presence of family members who receive the necessary training by the nurse and are more motivated, can separate the patient more easily and effectively from device help.

In addition, the presence of the family can also be effective in preventing the complications of diseases. For example, Maria Deja et al. (2006) conducted a quasi-experimental study in 2006 to investigate the effect of social support on mental functioning and the reduction of ARDS3 complications. For this study, they studied 35 patients with ARDS during their stay in the ICU and 6 months after discharge.

The results of the above study showed that in 29% of patients a significant reduction in ARDS complications and in 40% of cases a significant reduction in patients' mental complications was observed. (P <0.05).

PTSD, which can be one of the complications of hospitalization, plays an important role in delaying the patient's recovery. Early and timely rehabilitation can be effective in preventing PTSD. PTSD can prevent the patient from returning to normal life and community after the acute phase of the disease has passed. To combat and prevent this, rehabilitation measures should be started at the same time as hospitalization, as many brain functions may be irreversibly damaged during hospitalization.

For example, in a 2007 study of 100 ICU patients, Parthian Pendaripand et al. Found that delirium occurs in 73% of surgical patients and 63% of trauma patients admitted to the ICU, of which only 22% were able to return to their previous life after discharge. The results of the above study showed that these were 22% of those for whom rehabilitation had started during hospitalization. Various measures were taken for this rehabilitation, one of which was to increase the number of visits to family members and include the family in the patient rehabilitation program from the very beginning.

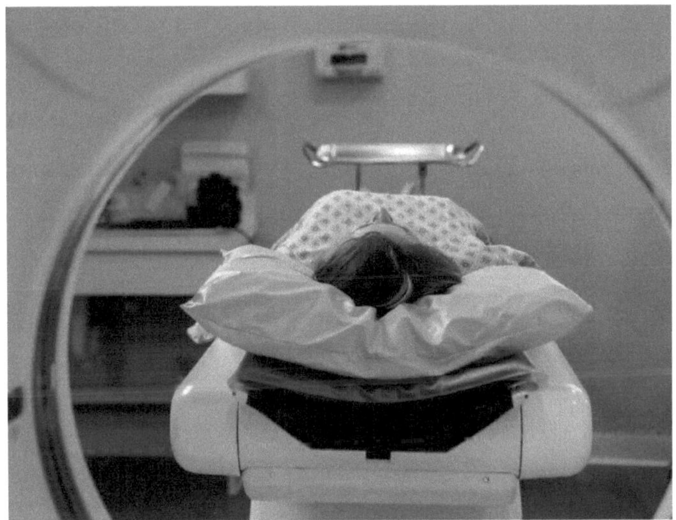

Figure 21. Midline Shift After Head Trauma

The absence and participation of the family in patient care causes great anxiety and stress for them, a large part of this is due to the nurses' belief in this regard. In this regard, Ghiasvandian et al. Conducted a quasi-experimental research study in 2010 with the aim of analyzing the effect of changing the open visit policy on nurses' beliefs about nursing care. In this study, due to opposition to large-scale appointment changes, a sample of 14 nurses working in the intensive care unit of a teaching hospital in Tabriz were selected, each of whom completed a researcher-made questionnaire twice. The questionnaire was designed with Likert scale and 28 questions about individual and social factors of nurses' beliefs about changing the visiting policy from limited to free. The results of the above study showed that the nurses' belief before the change in the appointment policy is negative, according to the criterion with a maximum score of 4, the average score was 76.71 ± 6.31 and after releasing the appointment, the average score was 79.64 ± 5.94. The difference in the distribution of nurses 'belief scores before and after the change of appointment policy was significant (P = 0.038), but the relationship between nurses' beliefs and social factors was not significant (P = 0.85). According to the findings of this study, the dominant factor in nurses' beliefs among social factors, especially the role of colleagues and supervisors and policy-making and management.

In line with the present study, the results of a study by Lautriti et al. (2007) in a 22-center RCT in France showed that providing a conference for the families of ICU patients, providing brochures about their condition, and attending the patient's bedside. Reduces their stress and anxiety. The rate of depression was also reduced in the experimental group compared to the control group. But the results of the study by Medlen et al. (1998) in a brief before and after study showed that nursing interventions such as a meeting with the family at the time of patient admission, preparation of an ICU booklet for the family and limited visits with the patient had an effect on overall satisfaction. He did not have a family. Registration of only 30 participants may have limited the power of this study. Consistent with the present study, the results of McCromick et al.'s (2010) study showed that meeting the material and spiritual needs of ICU patients' families can resolve inter-family conflicts and increase family awareness that talking or touching a loved one can be very helpful and help in how to control the symptoms of aggression and anxiety.

Therefore, based on these results, it can be said that family members are usually more stressed, anxious and anxious at the beginning of the ICU, perhaps the most important reason is the sudden and unexpected reaction to something that has happened.

As most patients were admitted to the ICU following an accident or other unforeseen event, and the family was more concerned about losing them than ever before, but the decline in GHQ scores in both groups showed over time. In fact, the reaction of family members to the hospitalization of a member in the ICU follows the steps of reacting to other tragic events. However, considering that the average GHQ score in the experimental group is lower than the control group, it can be stated that the presence of family members on the patient's bedside can play a significant role in his faster adaptation to the accident and gaining a sense of calm. This is because the general health of the family may be compromised by concerns about the patient's condition, feelings of inadequacy to save the patient, and lack of confidence in the proper and adequate care of the patient by staff. This problem sometimes manifests itself in the form of aggression, protests against staff and complaints to superiors. But being at the patient's bedside can go a long way in relieving these worries and helping to calm people down.

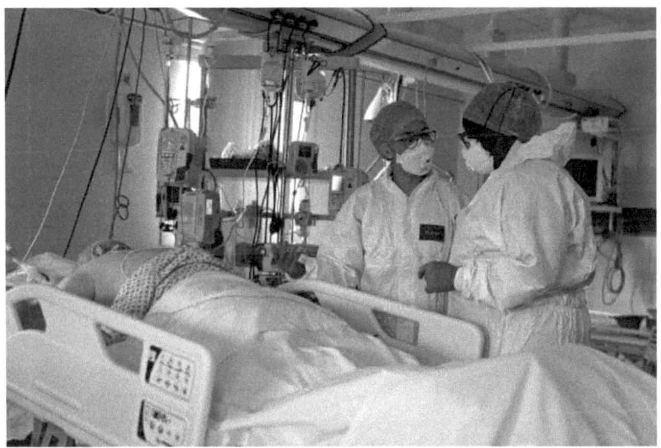

Figure 22. Tears were running all over my face': ICU medics on caring for Covid-19 patients

Bedside application

The results of research have shown that nurses can participate in patient care with adequate training of family members and plan treatment and diagnostic decisions with their presence. This can largely dispel misconceptions about family involvement in patient care, admission to the ICU, and how nurses care for the patient, and help improve communication in the ICU.

Application in education

The results of this study showed that the topics of sensory deprivation, the effect of sensory stimulation and the role and needs of ICU patients' families can be included in the topics and emphasized more.

Application in medical treatment policy

The results of the study indicate the positive effect of sensory stimulation by family members on improving the level of consciousness of coma patients and reducing their length of hospital stay in the ICU. Also, the presence of family members on the patient's bedside largely alleviates their worries and helps to calm them down and adapt to the accident faster.

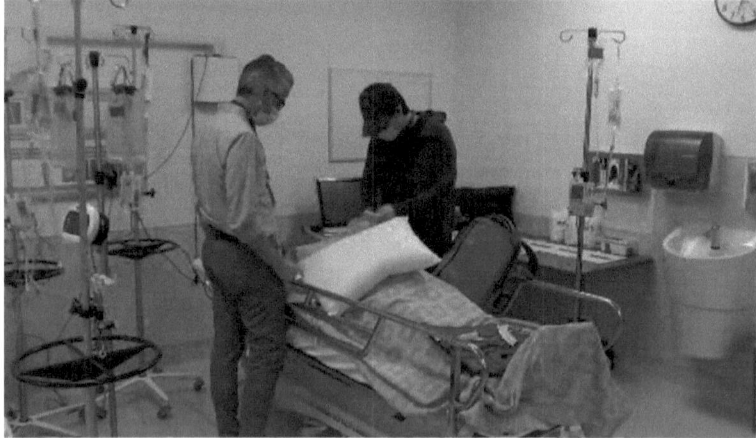

Figure 23. Toronto hospital trains doctors as ICU nurses to solve staff shortage

Therefore, it is suggested that in the treatment and care policies announced by health care decision makers, measures should be considered to enable family members to visit the patient by educating them in ICU wards, and forbidden visitation in these wards should be replaced. Give limited and principled meetings. Nurses in these wards, with adequate training, implement the sensory stimulation program as an essential part of care and nursing duties for the patient.

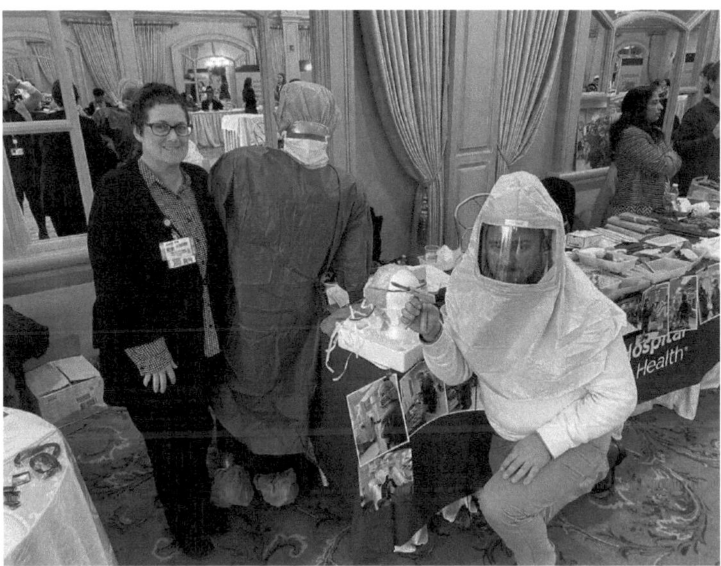

Figure 24. Students and Internships Archives

Chapter III

Nursing in Shock in ICU

What is Shock?

Shock is a condition in which systemic blood pressure is insufficient to carry oxygen and nutrients to vital organs and cell function. Shock is divided into 3 main categories:

- **Hypovolemic shock:** is caused by an insufficient volume of circulating blood, which can occur for reasons such as bleeding, burns, and dehydration. Hypovolemic shock is the most common type of shock.
- **Cardiogenic shock:** occurs due to inadequacy of the heart's pumping power due to dysfunction of the heart muscle.
- **Distributed shock:** is caused by a change in vascular tone that causes the size of the arteries to increase without increasing the volume of circulating blood. Anaphylactic shock (hypersensitivity reaction that leads to extensive dilation of systemic arteries), neurological shock (difficulty controlling the nervous system of blood vessels, especially following spinal cord injuries), and septic shock (release of vasoactive material in infections) are the three main categories of shock. They are distributive.

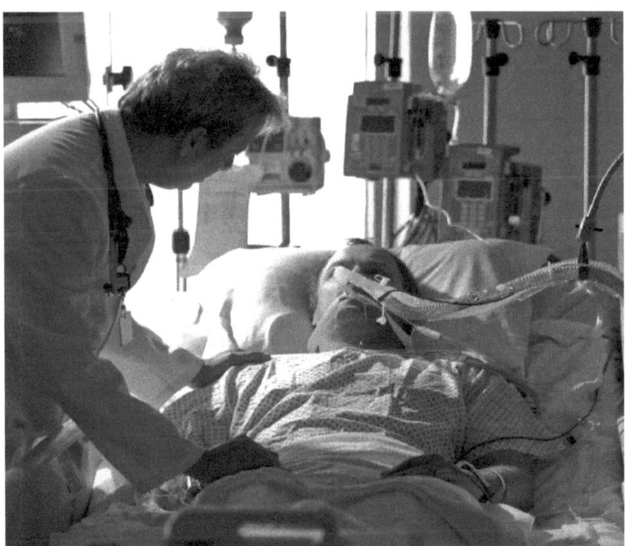

Figure 25. Shock/Trauma and Respiratory ICUs

Some Notes

In order for a shock due to bleeding to occur, 500-1500 cc of circulating blood volume must be lost. In other words, if a person loses a large amount of blood all at once or in a short period of time, the symptoms of shock show much faster than a person who loses a large amount of blood in a short period of time. Because of this, the range of circulating blood loss for shock varies from 500 to 1500 cc.

Shock in burns occurs due to the shift of plasma from the intravascular space to the interstitial space and the secretion of myocardial inhibitor (MDF), resulting in impaired cardiac output. In cases such as nephrotic syndrome, extreme hunger, surgery, severe trauma injuries, liver cirrhosis, pancreatitis, and intestinal obstruction, fluid shifts occur, which can lead to shock.

In addition to MI, other disorders such as large pulmonary embolism, pericardial tamponade, and compressive pneumothorax can lead to cardiogenic shock. If, for any reason, systemic blood pressure is not enough to nourish the tissues, the body uses compensatory mechanisms. It should be noted that these compensatory mechanisms are responsive only in the initial (compensatory) stage of shock, and if left untreated, it no longer responds to the body's needs, the later stages of shock begin.

The decrease in blood pressure is felt by pressure receptors (baroreceptors) located in the carotid sinus and aortic arch, and sends excitation waves to the sympathetic nerve centers in the medulla of the brain, which leads to the secretion of catecholamine's. Also in the aortic arch and carotid bodies, there are chemical receptors that are sensitive to lowering the pH and increasing the $paco_2$, leading to an increase in the number and depth of respiration and heart rate. However, all of these receptors and hormones are there to maintain moderate arterial pressure. Medium arterial pressure (MAP) is the median effective pressure that pushes blood forward in systemic organs. If the MAP is not at the normal level close to it (70-105 mmHg), tissue blood supply will not take place. The following formula can be used to obtain the approximate amount of MAP:

MAP: (systolic + 2 diastolic) divided by 3

Shock stages

1- **Non-advanced (compensatory) stage:** In this stage, also called the "fight or flight" response, the heart rate decreases slightly, but compensatory mechanisms can maintain blood pressure at or near normal blood flow. Maintain tissue to vital organs.

2- **Advanced stage:** In this stage, compensatory mechanisms are no longer sufficient. With continued vasoconstriction; The supply of oxygenated blood to the tissues is reduced as a result of anaerobic metabolism. As a result of anaerobic metabolism, lactic acidosis occurs, which causes very small arteries to dilate, reducing venous return and eventually oxygenated re-circulation. In addition, lactic acidosis increases capillary permeability and relaxes capillary sphincters. The looseness of the sphincters increases the pressure inside the capillaries, which together with the increase in capillary permeability causes fluid to leave the intravascular space and return to the tissues. This causes the formation of blood pools in the bed of small arteries, resulting in increased pressure and intravascular space.

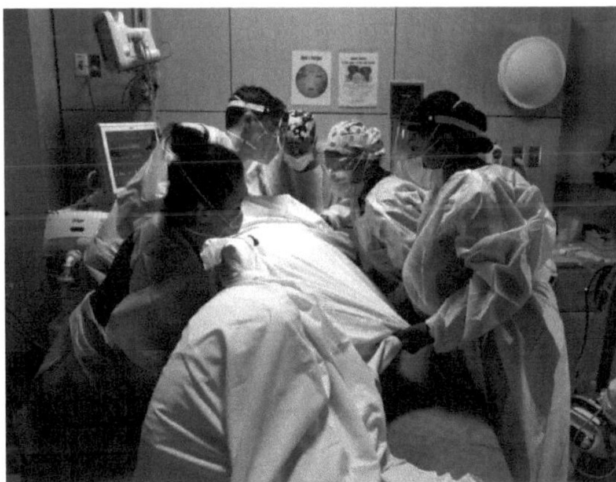

Figure 26. ICU Nurses Have Quit Because of The Stress Of COVID-19 Surge

Increased vascular capacity, decreased blood volume, and decreased cardiac function all reduce MAP, which lowers the pressure gradient for venous return to the heart, which in turn contributes to pool formation, decreased venous return, and decreased cardiac output. Although at this stage, all organs suffer from decreased blood flow, they prolong the following two events of shock syndrome: First, increased cardiac output causes ischemia and accumulation of chemical mediators. This can cause a heart pump to fail, even if it does not cause a heart attack.

The second event is a decrease in the self-regulatory function of microcirculation in response to a number of biochemical mediators released from the cell, thereby increasing capillary permeability, with tissue contraction compromising the arteries and veins. At this stage, the patient's prognosis worsens. Looseness of the pre-capillary sphincters causes fluid to leak from the capillaries, causing interstitial edema, and then reduced fluid return to the heart. Even if the cause of the shock is eliminated, the circulatory system itself causes the shock to last longer and creates a vicious cycle.

Finally, if the underlying cause of the shock is not eliminated, a regular sequence of compensatory responses continues in cycles, which are created in response to a decrease in tissue perfusion in the shock and are repeated over and over again.

3- **Irreversible stage:** This stage occurs if the defective cycle of insufficient blood supply to the tissue is not stopped. At this stage, the shock, despite the severity of the underlying cause, progresses increasingly, leading to cellular ischemia and necrosis leading to organ failure and death. At this stage, the duration of the shock is prolonged and the damage to the limbs is so severe that the patient does not respond to treatment and cannot survive. Despite treatment, blood pressure remains low. Following renal and hepatic insufficiency, toxic compounds are released from necrotic tissue and then severe metabolic acidosis develops. Anaerobic metabolism worsens acidosis by producing lactic acid. ATP stores are almost completely depleted and the mechanisms involved in energy storage are disrupted. Dysfunction of various organs has progressed to organ failure, in which case death is imminent. Clinical manifestations of shock: The table below briefly compares the clinical signs of different stages of shock.

Table 1. Clinical Signs of Shock Stages

Irreversible stage	Progressive stage	Compensatory stage
Requires mechanical or medical support	Systole less than 90-80 mmHg	Normal blood pressure
More than 150 times per minute, irregular or asystole	Heart rate more than 100 beats per minute	Heart rate more than 100 beats per minute
Requires endotracheal intubation	Fast and superficial, Crackle	Breathing: more than 20 times a minute
Yellow	Has petticoat	Cold, viscous and moist skin
Requires dialysis	Less than 0.5 mm / kg / h	Decreased urinary output
Loss of consciousness	Drowsiness	State of consciousness: Confusion
Severe acidosis	Metabolic acidosis	Respiratory alkalosis base acid balance

Clinical manifestations of shock in different systems

Respiratory system: tachypnea (rapid and shallow breathing) and respiratory alkalosis, pulmonary crackers, pulmonary edema.

Cardiovascular device: tachycardia, weak pulse and thread, hypotension, especially systolic pressure in the chest.

Nervous system - Endocrinology: Anxiety, anger and irritability (epinephrine secretion and overactive sympathetic activity), confusion, fainting and unconsciousness, cold and wet skin and dilated pupils.

Renal system: Decreased urinary output.

Gastrointestinal tract and liver: Bloody diarrhea (necrosis of the intestinal mucosa), bloody vomiting (stomach bleeding). Gastrointestinal ischemia can cause the release of bacterial toxins and their entry into the bloodstream. Due to the reduced function of the liver to filter bacteria, a person's susceptibility to infection increases. Liver enzymes increase and the person turns yellow. As the liver's ability to metabolize ammonia and lactic acid decreases, the effects of these substances on various systems also increase. Nausea and vomiting and decreased bowel sounds are other symptoms of shock.

Hematological system: Increased susceptibility to thrombosis Eventually the occurrence of DIC, which manifests itself as ecchymosis and petechiae in the skin (slow movement of blood in the capillaries, bacterial endotoxins and erythrocyte thromboplastin cause DIC).

Note: The elderly may take medications such as beta-blockers (to treat HNT), which mask tachycardia (the initial compensatory response to shock). The heart of the elderly may also react dysrhythmically to decreased myocardial oxygenation. Changes in mental status in the elderly may also be mistaken for part of the dementia process.

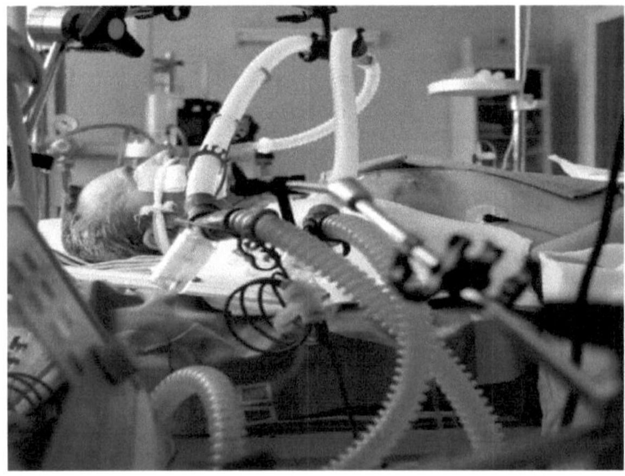

Figure 27. Critical Care Nursing Online

Chapter IV

Types of Shocks

Types of shocks

Shock can be classified according to the components of the perfusion in the following order:

1- Hypovolemic shock: is related to the loss of circulating fluid volume and in trauma injuries is mainly hemorrhagic. This type of shock is the most common type of trauma injury.

2- Distributed (or vasogenic) shock: is related to impaired vascular tone caused by several different causes.

3- Cardiogenic shock: is related to the dysfunction of the heart pump.

The most common cause of shock in a trauma victim is hemorrhagic or bleeding shock, and in dealing with a traumatized shock victim it should always be considered hemorrhagic unless proven otherwise.

Comparison of different types of shock

Hypovolemic	Hypotension, tachycardia Weak thready pulse Cool, pale, moist skin U/O decreased	Decreased CO Increased SVR
Cardiogenic	Hypotension, tachycardia Weak thready pulse Cool, pale, moist skin U/O < 30 ml/hr Crackles, tachypnea	Decreased CO Increased SVR
Neurogenic	Hypotension, BRADYCARDIA **WARM DRY SKIN**	Decreased CO **Venous & arterial vasodilation, loss sympathetic tone**
Anaphylactic	Hypotension, tachycardia Cough, dyspnea Pruritus, urticaria Restlessness, decreased LOC	Decreased CO Decreased SVR
Septic	Hypotension, Tachycardia Full bounding pulse, tachypnea **Pink, warm, flushed skin**	**Decreased** CO, **Decreased** SVR

Figure 28. Comparison of types of shocks

In general, the general signs and symptoms of shock include the following:

Following shock or hypoperfusion or inadequate tissue perfusion, it can rapidly affect systems of the body. These systems include the brain and central nervous system

(CNS), the heart and cardiovascular systems, the respiratory system, the skin and upper and lower limbs, and the kidneys. Therefore, the symptoms of hypoperfusion can include the following signs and symptoms:

Brain system and CNS: change in level of consciousness, anxiety, mental disorder, aggression and strange behavior. The victim suffers from shock due to cerebral ischemia and insufficient oxygen supply to the brain, suffering from anxiety, restlessness, and aggression. The victim is hungry for air and feels the need for more ventilation. The presence of a mask on the nose and mouth is considered as an obstacle for the injured person to breathe. This indicates insufficient oxygen supply and hypoxia. Detection of oxygen depletion with the help of a pulse oximetry device raises this suspicion. Saturation less than 95% is considered dangerous and the search for the cause of the shock is mandatory.

Cardiovascular system: tachycardia, decreased systolic blood pressure and pulse pressure.

Respiratory system: shallow and rapid respiration: Anaerobic metabolism due to decreased cellular oxygenation increases lactic acid production. Hydrogen ions from hypoxic acidosis stimulate the respiratory center and increase the number and depth of ventilation. So tachypnea is usually one of the first signs of shock. In the initial assessment there is no opportunity to count the number of breaths. Instead, it can be said that the number of breaths is low, normal, high or very high. Low respiration rate with shock indicates that the casualty is in deep shock and not far from cardiac arrest. Any high number of breaths is a cause for concern and is considered a pressure factor to find the cause of the shock.

Upper and lower skin and limbs: Cold, pale and moist skin, sweating and even cyanosis with increased capillary bruising time (cyanotic) or its point in hypovolemic shock, the reason for hemoglobin lack of oxygen and lack of oxygen supply to peripheral tissues. Pale skin, cyanotic or spotty do not get enough blood due to one of the underlying factors.

- Contraction of peripheral arteries (often associated with hypovolemia).
- Insufficient number of RBCs.
- Cut off blood flow to a part of the body such as what might happen in a fracture.

Note: Cyanosis may not be seen in casualties who have lost a significant number of their RBCs due to bleeding and have hypoxia. In black people, cyanosis may be found on the lips, gums and palms.

Skin temperature: When the body shifts blood from the skin to more important areas, the skin temperature drops. If the skin temperature is cold to the touch, it is a sign that either perfusion of the skin has decreased or energy production is having problems and shock has occurred.

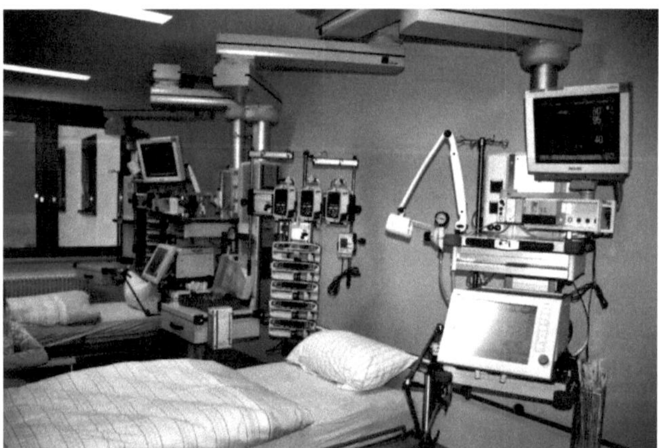

Figure 29. Intensive care unit

Capillary filling time: The capillary filling time test has recently been evaluated as a poor test in shock diagnosis. However, this test is more of a capillary bed perfusion adequacy test and less of a shock detection test. However, one of the causes of prolonged capillary filling time is decreased cardiac output due to hypovolemia. This test is a useful diagnostic marker in hypovolemic shock along with other symptoms and can help emergency technicians review care and rescue measures. Some factors such as age, pregnancy, underlying diseases, medication use and exercise status can affect the onset of signs and symptoms of shock and disrupt the assessment process.

Age: Injuries at both ends of the life line, infants and the elderly, have little protection against acute bleeding and shock. Therefore, a small injury in these people may cause irreversible shock. On the other hand, children and adolescents have a very high compensatory power against bleeding and may seem relatively normal at first glance. A closer examination of these people can show signs of shock such as mild tachycardia and tachypnea, pale skin, delayed capillary filling, and anxiety. Due to their powerful compensatory mechanisms, children are in a deadly emergency situation if they are in the non-compensatory phase. Older people are more sensitive to some of the consequences of long-term shock, such as acute renal failure (ARF).

Pregnancy: In pregnant women, blood volume may increase by up to 50%. Heart rate and cardiac output also increase. For this reason, during pregnancy, a pregnant woman may not show signs of shock until she has lost 30 to 35 percent of her blood volume. Also in the third trimester of pregnancy, the uterus can compress the inferior vena cava, reduce venous return to the heart, and cause hypotension. This condition can be counteracted by lifting the injured person to the right after immobilizing the backboard. If the hypotension continues with this maneuver, it indicates dangerous bleeding.

Underlying diseases: Injured people with underlying diseases such as coronary artery disease and chronic obstructive pulmonary disease (COPD) usually have less compensatory power against bleeding and shock. These people may develop angina due to an increased heart rate. Injuries that have an artificial pacemaker are not able to produce the compensatory tachycardia that is required to maintain blood pressure.

Taking Medications: Taking certain medications disrupts the body's compensatory mechanisms. Beta-blockers and calcium blockers, which are used to treat high blood pressure, prevent compensatory tachycardia in order to maintain blood pressure. Nonsteroidal anti-inflammatory drugs (NSAIDs), which are used to treat arthritis and musculoskeletal pain, can interfere with platelet activity and blood clotting, leading to increased bleeding.

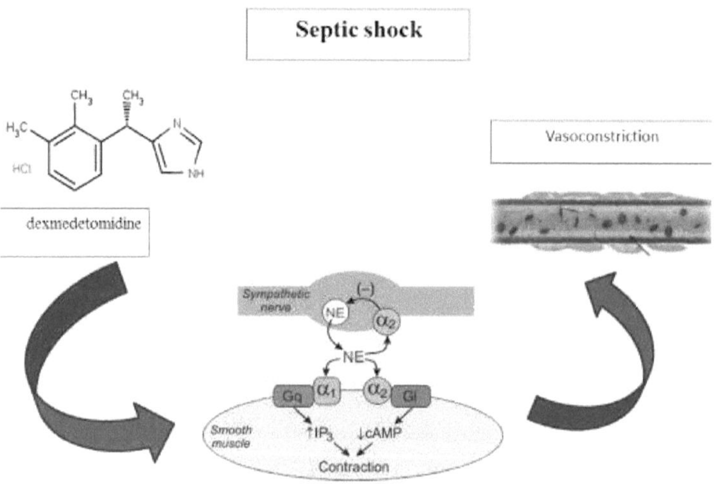

Figure 30. Evaluating the Effect of Dexmedetomidine on Hemodynamic Status of Patients with Septic Shock

Exercise status: Professional athletes usually have a high compensatory capacity. Many of them have a resting heart rate of about 40 to 50 beats per minute. Therefore, the presence of a heart rate of 100 to 110 beats per minute or hypotension in a professional athlete indicates significant bleeding in this person.

Shock effects

If people with persistent shock are not treated well, they will suffer from several complications. For this reason, immediate diagnosis and rapid response to shock are essential.

- Acute renal failure
- Acute Respiratory Distress Syndrome (ARDS)
- Hematological insufficiency
- Liver failure
- Multiple organ failure

Hypovolemic shock

It is a condition in which, for various reasons, the volume of fluid in the circulation decreases. As a result, it leads to insufficient perfusion at the tissue level. Inadequate perfusion then reduces oxygenation at the cellular level, causes cellular anaerobic metabolism and accumulation of harmful substances in the tissue, and if not treated in time, cell and organ death occurs. When the volume of blood suddenly decreases due to dehydration (loss of plasma) or due to bleeding (loss of plasma and RBCs), the relationship between fluid volume and the size of the vascular capacity becomes unbalanced. The size of the vascular capacity is still normal but the volume of fluid has decreased. Hypovolemic shock is the most common type of shock in prehospital conditions and bleeding is the most common cause in trauma patients.

When blood leaves the circulation, the heart is stimulated to increase its flow. This stimulation, which is caused by the release of epinephrine from the adrenal gland, increases the number and contractile strength of the heart. The sympathetic nervous system also releases epinephrine, which causes blood vessels to constrict. As a result, the size of the vascular capacity is somewhat reduced and is proportional to the amount of fluid remaining.

Vascular contraction leads to the closure of peripheral capillaries and changes from aerobic to anaerobic at the cellular level of metabolism. These compensatory mechanisms work well together to some extent. When other defense mechanisms cannot overcome the reduction in blood volume, the injured person's blood pressure decreases. Decreased blood pressure indicates that the shock has become compensatory to non-compensatory, with symptoms of imminent death. The injured person who shows signs of compensation is already in a state of shock and is not on the verge of going to shock. Unless immediate rescue measures are taken, the casualty in the irreversible shock is only one step away from the final ceiling of death.

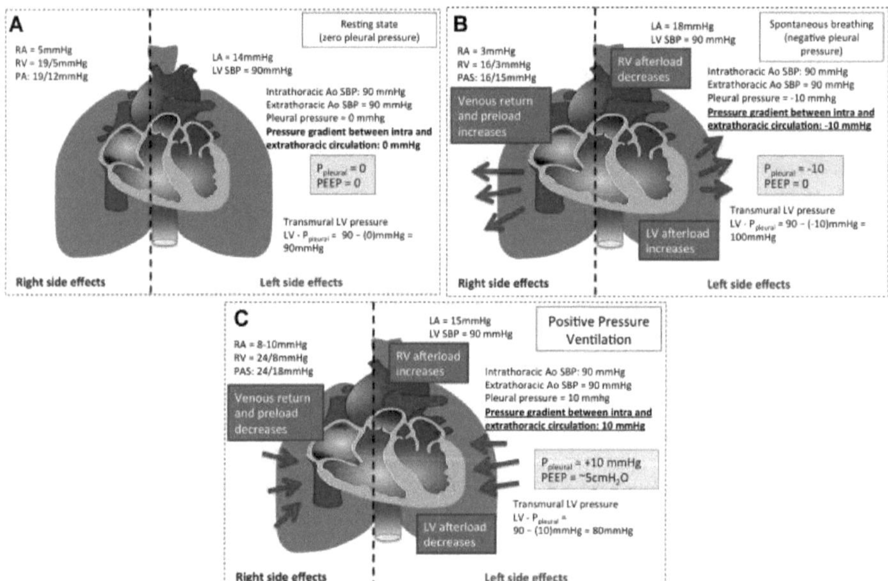

Figure 31. Positive Pressure Ventilation in Cardiogenic Shock: Review of the Evidence and Practical Advice

Stages of hypovolemic shock

1- Compensated shock

It is the initial stage of shock during which the body is still able to meet its basic metabolic needs by relying on a set of compensatory functions. These progressive compensatory processes cause a set of signs and symptoms that include:

- Pulse rate increases
- Pulse power decreases
- The skin becomes cold and paste
- Anxiety, restlessness and aggression increase
- Thirst, fatigue and air hunger occur.

2- Uncompensated shock

It starts when the compensatory mechanisms can no longer respond to the lost blood or maintain preload. The mechanisms that initially compensated for the lost blood have now failed and the body is rapidly collapsing. Entry into irreversible shock is characterized by the following symptoms:

- The pulse becomes untouchable.
- Blood pressure drops with a steep slope.
- The patient loses consciousness.
- Breathing slows down or stops.

3- Irreversible shock

Occurs when the body's cells are so damaged and dead that organs are unable to perform their normal functions. Although good resuscitation can restore blood pressure and pulse, organ failure will eventually lead to the death of the organism. It is very difficult to detect the passage to the irreversible stage of shock in the scene. What is clear is that the longer a patient stay in the irreversible shock phase, the more likely he or she is to enter the irreversible shock phase.

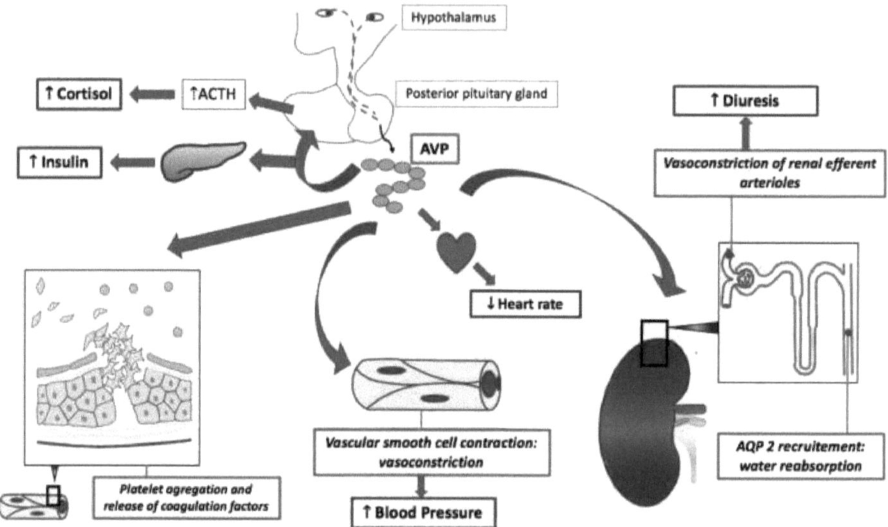

Figure 32. Vasopressin and its analogues in shock states

Hemorrhagic shock

On average, a 70 kg adult has about 5 liters of blood in his circulatory system. Hemorrhagic shock (hypovolemic shock due to bleeding) can be classified into four categories based on the severity and amount of bleeding. This category is related to the volume of blood lost in acute bleeding and its associated signs and symptoms. It should be noted that each person's response to blood loss varies according to the speed and progression of the disease. The use of these categories helps emergency personnel determine the relative severity of blood loss and the need for immediate intervention.

Category I bleeding

Loss of about 15% (> 750CC) of body blood in adults in which the body's compensatory mechanism is mediated by vascular contraction.

in this case:

Consciousness: The patient is alert and may be a little anxious.

Pulse: Peripheral pulses are quite palpable.

Heart rate: May increase slightly.

Systolic blood pressure: Normal.

Breathing rate: Normal.

Skin condition: Normal.

Bleeding Category II

Loss of about 15-30% (750-1500cc) of body blood in which the body's compensatory mechanism is impaired by vasoconstriction and blood flow is diverted to vital organs. in this case:

State of consciousness: Anxiety and confusion, accompanied by increased cerebral hypoxia.

Radial pulse: Probably weak.

Heart rate: Looking for a sympathetic response, tachycardia and usually above 100 beats per minute.

Systolic blood pressure: A decrease or increase in systolic blood pressure occurs. Lowering systolic blood pressure may occur without changing diastolic blood pressure, resulting in a narrow pulse pressure.

Respiratory rate: Following sympathetic stimulation, the respiratory rate increases and the patient has tachypnea.

Skin condition: Pale, cold and moist.

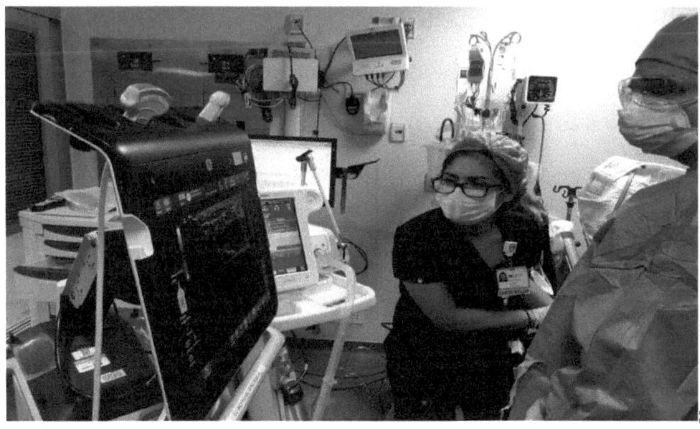

s

Figure 33. Diary of a COVID-19 nurse: Exhaustion, teamwork, struggle and celebration

Category III bleeding

Loss of about 30-40% (1500-2000cc) of body blood in which compensatory mechanisms (vasoconstriction) are reduced and not tolerated. Cardiac output is reduced and life-threatening. in this case:

Consciousness: The patient is confusing, drowsy, and possibly unresponsive.

Pulse: Peripheral pulses are eliminated.

Heart rate: Looking for a sympathetic response, tachycardia and usually above 120 beats per minute.

Systolic blood pressure: A decrease in systolic blood pressure below 90 mm Hg occurs.

Respiratory rate: Following sympathetic stimulation, respiratory rate increases.

Skin condition: The color is gray and completely cold and moist.

Note: In class 3 bleeding, symptoms of hypovolemic shock are seen.

Category IV bleeding

More than 40% (more than 2000cc) of body blood is lost. Compensatory contraction itself is impaired and causes further destruction of blood supply to tissues and oxygen delivery, in which the patient is drowsy, lethargic, and has decreased level of consciousness. Clear symptoms of shock are seen. in this case:

Consciousness: The patient is unconscious

Pulse: It is also difficult to touch the central carotid and femoral pulses.

Heart rate: progresses to severe bradycardia.

Systolic blood pressure: There is a severe drop in blood pressure.

Respiration rate: Rapid, shallow and ineffective breathing.

Skin condition: The skin becomes blemished.

Note that in class 4 bleeding, the symptoms of hypovolemic shock are clearly visible.

Note: Circulating blood volume in children is 75-80 ml / kg. And because the blood volume of children is much smaller than that of adults, the loss of a small amount of blood may be significant in terms of hemodynamic effects. In children with shock, first cardiac output and blood pressure are maintained at normal levels through compensatory mechanisms such as vasoconstriction, tachycardia, and increased cardiac contractility. In fact, hypotension is not seen in children with trauma until the volume of blood that has been acutely lost reaches about 25-30% of the circulating blood volume. Therefore, the presence of normal blood pressure does not rule out the presence of shock. Hypotension is a sign of a serious condition and indicates that cardiovascular failure has occurred and cardiovascular arrest is imminent.

	On presentation and admission to Emergency department (ED)	15 minutes after admission	30 minutes after admission	45 minutes after admission	60 minutes after admission
1. Heart rate (bpm)	130	120	110	100	94
2. BP (mm Hg)	90/60	100/60	110/70	120/80	120/80
3. Pulse pressure (mm Hg)	30	40	40	40	40
4.Respiratory rate (breaths/min)	32	28	24	19	18
5.Urine output (ml/hr)	12				24
6.Neurological status (GCS = Glasgow Coma Scale)	13	13	15	15	15
7. Base deficit	8				5

Figure 34. Evaluation and management of haemorrhagic shock in polytrauma: Clinical practice guidelines

Distributed or vasogenic shock

In distributed or vasogenic shock, unlike hypovolemic shock, we do not experience hypovolemia due to bleeding, vomiting, or diarrhea, but in this type of shock, resistance to blood flow decreases because the size of blood vessels increases for various reasons. This decrease in resistance reduces diastolic blood pressure. If this decrease in resistance is accompanied by a decrease in cardiac output, cardiac output will also be reduced, resulting in a drop in systolic and diastolic blood pressure.

Distributed shock can be caused by a loss of control of the autonomic nervous system over the smooth muscles in the walls of blood vessels, as well as the release of chemicals that cause vasodilation. This lack of control can be due to trauma to the spinal cord (neurogenic shock), severe infection (septic shock), allergic reactions (anaphylactic shock), or even stimulation of the parasympathetic system (vasovagal shock) may occur. Coping with this type of shock is improving blood oxygenation and maintaining the flow of blood to the brain and vital organs.

Neurogenic shock

Neurogenic shock occurs following damage to the spinal cord and disruption of the sympathetic system. In the spinal cord, this injury is usually related to the thoracolumbar region. Due to the loss of sympathetic control over the muscles in the peripheral artery wall, the arteries below the affected area become vasodilated. Also, due to the lack of coping with parasympathetic activity on the heart, there is usually bradycardia instead of tachycardia. This severe decrease in vascular resistance and peripheral vasodilation leads to relative hypovolemia and eventually hypotension. It should be noted that this peripheral vasodilation and bradycardia can last for several days.

Symptoms of neurogenic shock

- We have a decrease in systolic and diastolic blood pressure.
- Pulse pressure is normal.
- We usually have a decrease in heart rate or bradycardia.
- Pulse quality may be poor.
- We have hot and dry skin, especially under the affected area.
- The casualty is conscious, unless he has a traumatic brain injury.
- Loss of sensory and motor reflexes

Note that casualties with neurogenic shock may also have other bleeding injuries. Therefore, people with neurogenic shock with symptoms of hypovolemia, such as tachycardia, should be treated appropriately.

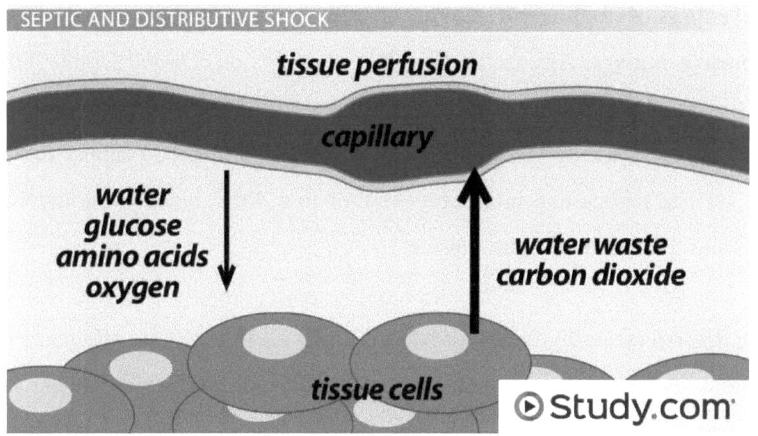

Figure 35. Hypovolemic Shock Symptoms, Causes, and Treatment

Vasovagal or psychogenic shock

Vasovagal or psychogenic shock is usually caused by involvement of the parasympathetic nervous system. Stimulation of the vagus nerve (tenth cranial nerve) causes bradycardia. Increased parasympathetic activity leads to temporary peripheral vasodilation and hypotension. If bradycardia and vasodilation are severe, cardiac output is significantly reduced and cerebral blood flow is impaired. Vasovagal syncope (fainting) occurs when the patient loses consciousness. This vasodilation and bradycardia in psychogenic shock is limited to a few minutes, and if the patient is placed in a horizontal position, normal blood pressure returns quickly. Because the vasovagal attack is self-limiting, it probably does not lead to shock, and the body quickly returns to normal before a systemic disturbance in the perfusion process occurs.

Cardiogenic shock

Cardiogenic shock is caused by the heart's inadequacy in pumping blood. This shock is caused by internal factors (due to heart damage) and external factors (due to external heart problem).

Internal causes of cardiogenic shock

Heart muscle damage: Any factor that affects the function or blood supply of the heart muscle (myocardium) and weakens it can reduce cardiac output and cause cardiogenic shock. These factors may be due to a sudden cessation of blood supply to the heart muscle, such as myocardial infarction (MI), or to a direct blow to the myocardium, such as blunt trauma to the heart muscle.

Cardiac disorders: Arrhythmias, or heart disorders, can affect the efficiency of heart contractions and lead to impaired cardiac output and cardiogenic shock. Because cardiac output is the product of the number of heart beats per minute multiplied by the stroke volume (CO = PR * SV), any irregularity that leads to a decrease in the number of beats or a shortening of the ventricular filling time (which reduces the stroke volume) Disrupts cardiac output. Hypoxia and blunt trauma to the heart are among the most common causes of cardiac abnormalities and arrhythmias such as premature ventricular contraction (PVC) and tachycardia.

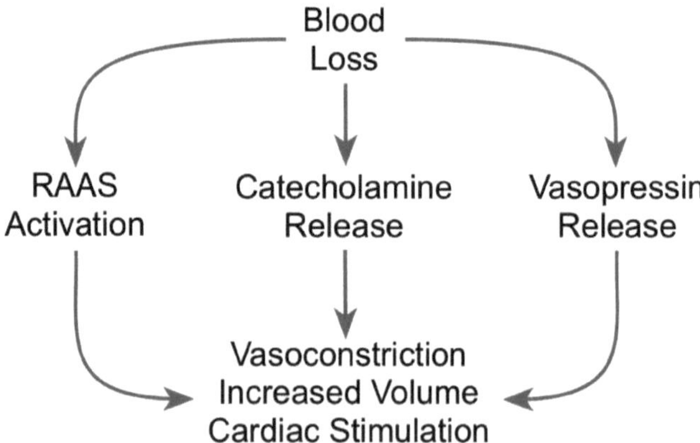

Figure 36. CV Physiology, Hemorrhagic Shock

Valvular heart injuries: Compressive and strong injuries to the chest area can cause damage and rupture of the heart muscles. These valvular injuries may lead to acute regurgitation. In this case, a significant amount of blood returns to the cavity from which it was pumped. This condition leads to congestive heart failure (CHF) and manifests as cardiogenic shock and pulmonary edema.

External causes of cardiogenic shock

Cardiac tamponade: The presence of excess fluid in the pericardial sac can prevent the heart from filling completely in the diastolic phase and reduce cardiac output. According to Starling's law, incomplete filling reduces the heart's contractile strength. In penetrating heart trauma, with each contraction, more blood enters the pericardial sac and impairs cardiac output. Continuation of this condition leads to severe cardiogenic shock and death.

Compression pneumothorax: Following compression pneumothorax, the mediastinum moves from the affected area to the opposite side. Compression and torsion of the superior and inferior vena cava veins, as well as increased pulmonary vascular resistance due to intrathoracic enlargement, cause severe impairment of venous return to the heart, resulting in a significant reduction in cardiac overload. Due to thc filling disorder, the heart loses its effective function as a pump and cardiogenic shock occurs immediately.

Septic shock

Septic shock or infectious shock is seen in patients with severe and dangerous infections, in this case; Cytokines, which are active local hormones produced by white blood cells in response to infections, damage the walls of blood vessels, resulting in peripheral vasodilation and leakage of fluid from the capillaries into the interstitial space. Thus, this type of shock has both distributive and hypovolemic shock characteristics. Cardiac output decreases due to vasodilation and fluid loss, and hypotension occurs when the heart is no longer able to compensate. Septic shock never really occurs within minutes, but prehospital technicians may be responsible for caring for a septic shock victim in inter-center transfer missions. People with gastrointestinal trauma who do not receive immediate medical attention also experience septic shock.

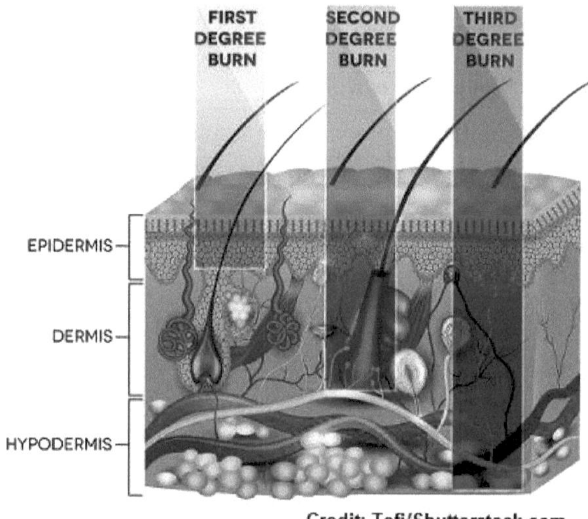

Figure 37. Hypovolemic Shock NCLEX

Chapter V

Shock Management in ICU

Shock Treatment and Nursing Care

A) General therapies

Shock treatment should be started in the presence of at least 2 of the following: systolic blood pressure, 80 mm Hg or less, pulse pressure of 20 mm Hg or less, and pulse rate greater than 120 min.

1- Elimination of the cause of the shock: Accurate examination and diagnosis of the main cause of the shock is the basis of treatment. Septic shock is more difficult to diagnose than shock. For example, if dehydration is caused by hyperglycemia, insulin is prescribed, and if diabetes is tasteless, desmopressin is prescribed.

2- Improve oxygenation: In all types of shock, supplemental oxygen is prescribed to protect the client from hypoxemia. In severe and prolonged stages of shock, intubation or tracheostomy is performed to relax a tired client (reduce respiratory work) or to correct respiratory failure. However, the goal of treatment is to maintain pao_2 and $o_2$sat above 90. Mechanical ventilation may be used to improve pulmonary ventilation.

3- Fluid replacement: Prescription fluids may be crystalloid, colloidal, or blood. Crystalloids are electrolyte fluids that move freely between the intravascular and interstitial spaces and can be isotonic, hypertonic, or hypotonic. Isotonic solutions with electrolyte concentrations similar to extracellular fluid are often used to treat shock. Crystalloid solutions include normal saline and ringer lactate (lactate to bicarbonate is effective in reducing acidosis). One of the disadvantages of isotonic crystalloid solutions is that about 2.3 of them enter the interstitial space and only 1.3 remain inside the arteries.

This causes fluid to accumulate in the extracellular space, causing more fluid to be injected than needed. During rapid infusion of crystalline isotonic fluid, be careful of edema, especially pulmonary, due to the entry of fluids into the interstitial spaces. To reduce the risk of pulmonary edema, in cases of severe hypovolemic shock, crystalloid hypertonic solutions such as 5% sodium chloride are used. High osmolality of these solutions causes the transfer of fluid from the intracellular space to the extracellular space, which means that less volume of fluid is needed to provide the appropriate intravascular volume. Heat disturbance noted. Do not prescribe lactate Ringer in cases where the patient has a hepatic impairment because the liver is unable to convert lactate to bicarbonate.

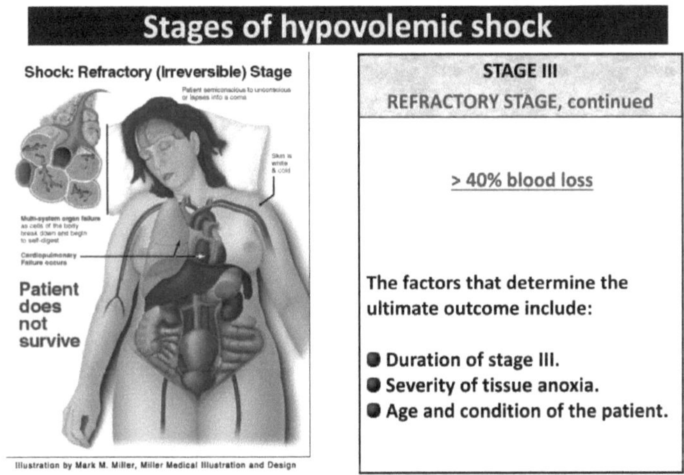

Figure 38. Cardiovascular Block Physiology Shock PowerPoint Presentation, free download

Colloidal solutions contain large plasma proteins that are unable to exit the capillary membrane and, through oncotic pressure, draw fluids from the interstitial space into the intravascular space. it is needed. Albumin is a colloidal solution made from donor blood plasma and is therefore heated to prevent the transmission of human disease. Because albumin may travel into the interstitial space in the lungs and draw water into the lungs, causing ARDS to develop, there is a problem with its use. Dextran is a synthetic colloidal solution. This solution can impair platelet adhesion, so it is not used in hypovolemic shock due to bleeding or coagulation disorders. Be careful of anaphylactic reactions when using colloidal solutions.

Hetastarch is another colloidal solution that lasts up to 36 hours but prolongs the flow and coagulation time. If bleeding is the primary cause of shock, large doses of compressed red blood cells or whole blood may be needed. Sugar serum should not be used to compensate for fluids because as dextrose is metabolized, the remaining hypotonic water causes more fluid shifts.

However, if any fluid is prescribed, the patient should be monitored for side effects. The most serious complication is increased cardiovascular load and pulmonary edema. Patients should be monitored for urinary outflow, changes in consciousness, skin perfusion, bulging vein bulging, and vital signs. Lung sounds, especially for the presence of crackles, should be checked. Central venous pressure (CVP) measurement is the most accurate way to check the adequacy of the volume of prescribed fluid, which normally has a range of 2-12 cm.

Fluids can be continued if the patient's CVP is low, the lungs are clean, and there are no signs of congestive heart failure. Hb, HCT, I.O, BUN, Cr and ABG are other parameters that must be controlled.

4- Vasoactive drugs (affecting blood vessels)

Vascular contractors: These drugs increase systemic blood pressure by contracting peripheral arterioles. The purpose of using these drugs is to maintain blood pressure in the range of 70-80 mm Hg for tissue blood supply, but increasing the pressure to more than this amount with these drugs is not reasonable because it leads to increased cardiac output and consequently increased heart rate. Reduces abdominal viscera. The use of vasoconstrictors in cardiogenic shock is prohibited.

Vascular dilators: Shock-induced vasoconstriction increases capillary pressure, facilitates fluid loss from the intravascular to interstitial space, changes in blood flow, especially to the abdominal organs, facilitates the accumulation of waste products, and impairs cell nutrition. Vascular dilators dilate the arteries of the heart, skeletal muscles, and bronchi, thereby reducing the preload and post load of the heart, and ultimately the workload of the heart, and reduce the effects of vasoconstriction. In hypovolemic shock, body fluids must be replenished before prescribing these drugs, because prescribing this drug, along with a lack of circulating blood volume, causes a drop in blood pressure. Clients treated with these drugs; it is better to sleep relatively straight to prevent hypotension.

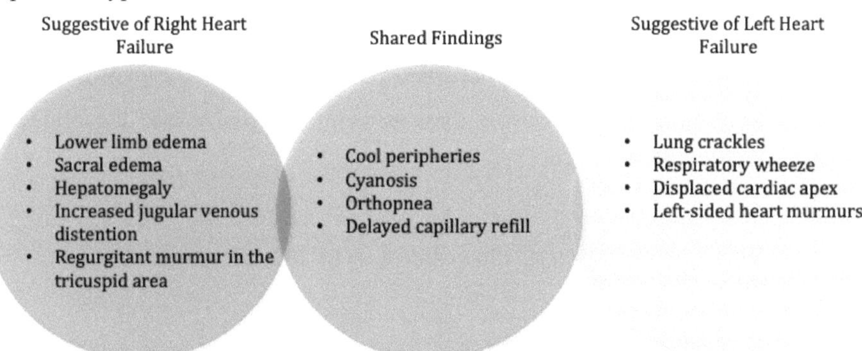

Figure 39. Cardiogenic Shock

Beta-1 receptor stimulants are another class of drugs that increase heart rate and myocardial contractility, and when taking effective vascular drugs, the patient's vital signs should be monitored every 15 minutes. It is best to administer these drugs through the central venous route because the release of some drugs from the vein can cause tissue necrosis. Vascular drugs should be discontinued gradually (every 15 minutes with blood pressure control) as abrupt discontinuation of these drugs causes severe hemodynamic instability and exacerbated shock.

5- Help blood circulation

Giving the patient a proper position: Trendlenberg's modified form (raising the legs by 30 to 45 degrees, straightening the torso, slightly raising the head and shoulders) is a major position in people with shock. This condition improves venous blood flow from the lower extremities without applying abdominal visceral pressure to the diaphragm. However, this position is not effective in severe hypovolemia and should not be used in people with cardiogenic shock due to increased cardiac output.

Shockproof pants: It is a garment that covers from the underside of the ribs to the ankles. The pressure from these pants increases vascular resistance and reduces the size of blood vessels in the abdomen and legs, which ultimately leads to resistance in the heart and increased arterial blood pressure. This device is often used in trauma situations outside the hospital. Due to the reduced blood supply to the lower extremities, which leads to acidosis in the pressed tissues, there are conflicting opinions about the use of these pants. The use of these pants is prohibited in case of cardiogenic shock.

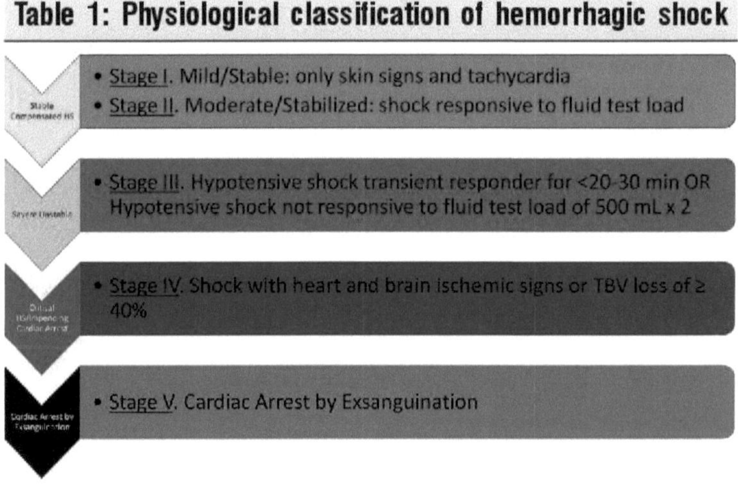

Figure 40. The Need for a Physiological Classification of Hemorrhagic Shock

6- Nutritional support: Increasing the speed of metabolism during shock increases the need for energy so that the patient needs more than 3000 calories per day. Lack of energy supply causes muscle mass to break down, even in the presence of high fat stores. Skeletal muscle resorption can prolong the healing process of shock. Intestinal or intravenous supportive feeding should be started as soon as possible. Glutamine (an essential amino acid in stress) must be supplied. It is a source of energy for lymphocytes and macrophages.

B) Therapeutic measures based on the type of shock

Hypovolemic shock

In this type of shock, the main goals of treatment are:

1- Maintain intravascular volume to prevent events that cause insufficient blood flow to the tissue.

2- Redistribute fluids by adjusting the Trendlenberg position.

3- Correction of factors involved in reducing the volume of fluids. However, fluid intake is an important part of treatment.

Cardiogenic shock

This shock mainly occurs in infarction of the anterior wall of the heart. Severe metabolic disorders (severe hypoxemia, acidosis, hypoglycemia, compression pneumothorax), cardiomyopathies, cardiac tamponade, and valvular disorders are other factors that cause cardiogenic shock. Due to impaired blood flow, the weakened tissue of the heart cannot move blood forward, and as a result, fluid accumulates in the lungs due to insufficient ventricular drainage during systole.

In addition to correcting the underlying factor, the first therapeutic measures in cardiogenic shock are:

- Giving oxygen
- Control chest pain
- Provide selected fluids
- Giving drugs that affect the arteries
- Controlling your heart rate by inserting a pacemaker or medication
- Relieve anxiety

In the early stages of shock, administering 2-6 liters of oxygen per minute through the nasal cannula can increase the oxygen saturation to 90%. Morphine is used to relieve pain. In addition to its analgesic properties, morphine increases the preload and post load of the heart by dilating the veins. Drugs commonly used to treat cardiogenic shock include dobutamine, nitroglycerin, and dopamine.

Dubotamine with its inotropic effect increases the intensity of heart muscle activity and thus increases cardiac output. It also reduces pulmonary and systemic vascular resistance by stimulating alpha receptors, thereby reducing cardiac overload and improving cardiac output. Nitroglycerin at low doses dilates the veins, thereby reducing the preload, and at high doses it dilates the arteries, reducing the back load. By these mechanisms, blood flow to the myocardial tissue also increases.

Dopamine is another low-dose drug that increases blood flow to the kidneys and prevents mesenteric ischemia. At moderate doses, it improves the contractile power of the heart and slightly increases the heart rate, so it improves the heart rate, and at high doses, it causes narrowing of the arteries, which increases the load on the heart, which is not a good effect. In severe metabolic acidosis, which occurs in the late stages of shock, the effectiveness of dopamine is reduced.

To maximize the effectiveness of any vasoactive drug, metabolic acidosis must be corrected. Diuretics are another class of drugs used to reduce the workload of the heart caused by fluid retention.

Antiarrhythmic drugs are also part of the treatment of cardiogenic shock. In cases where the cardiac output has not improved despite oxygen delivery, vasoactive drugs, and fluids, mechanical aids such as an intra-aortic balloon pump may be used temporarily to improve cardiac function. Hypoxia, electrolyte imbalances and acid-base disorders cause dangerous arrhythmias in patients with shock.

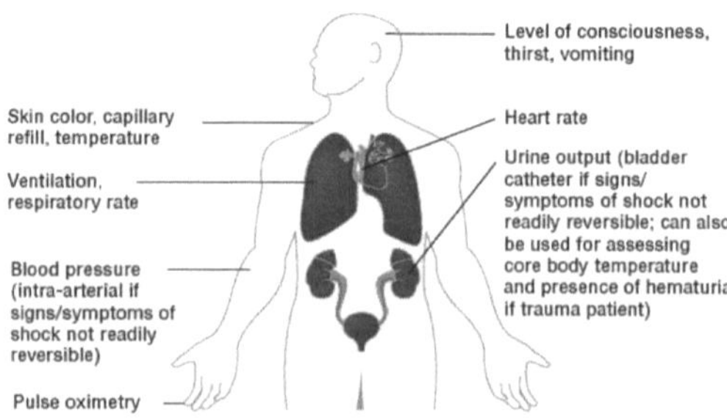

Figure 41. Hypovolemic Shock, Pharmacotherapy A Pathophysiologic Approach, 9th Ed.

Distributive shock

Septic shock: In the past, septic shock was believed to have two stages: The first stage is the hyper dynamic or warm stage, which is characterized by increased cardiac output and vasodilation. Blood pressure may remain within normal limits. The heart rate rises, causing tachycardia, and the patient's temperature rises to a fever, with hot, red skin and a full pulse. The number of breaths increases. Urinary incontinence may be reduced or remain normal. Manifested by impaired gastrointestinal tract with vomiting, diarrhea, and decreased intestinal sounds. The patient may show slight changes in state of consciousness, such as confusion or restlessness.

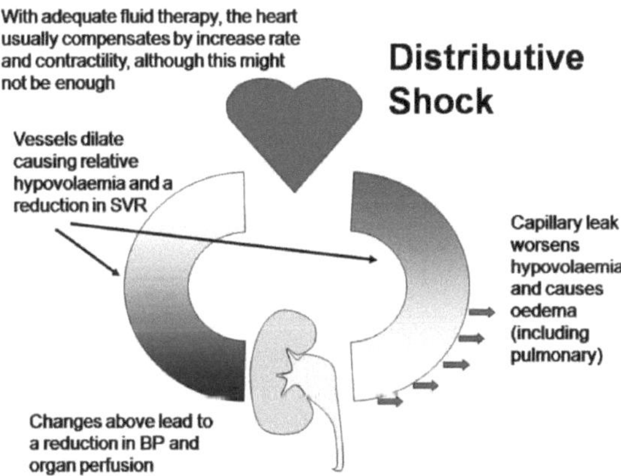

Figure 42. Distributive shock definition, causes, symptoms, diagnosis, treatment & prognosis

The next stage is the hypodynamic or irreversible stage, which is characterized by a decrease in cardiac output associated with vasoconstriction, indicating the body's attempt to compensate for hypovolemia due to loss of intravascular fluid due to capillary leakage. At this stage, blood pressure drops and the skin is cold and pale. The temperature may be normal or below normal. Heart rate and respiration remain high. Urinary production stops and multiple organ failure develops due to organ dysfunction. Rapid recovery of fluids, especially crystalloid fluids, is also a priority in this shock.

In addition to general therapies, therapeutic antibiotics are a major component of this type of shock (if the infectious agent is a bacterium). If there is not enough time for culture, treatment with broad-spectrum antibiotics is started. Drugs are also used to inhibit chemical mediators such as endotoxin or procalcitonin.

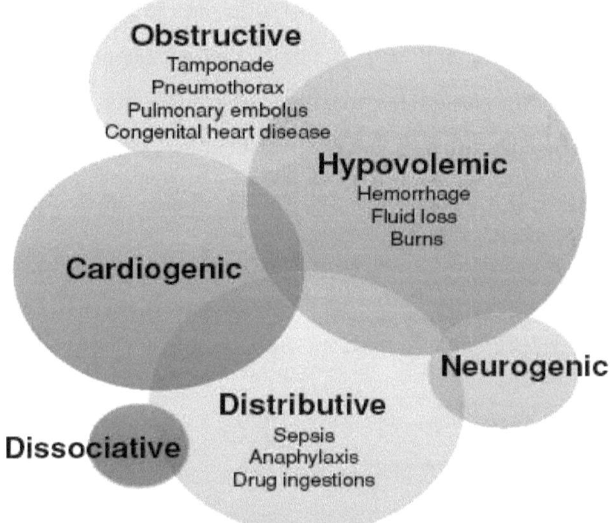

Figure 43. Shock, Anesthesia Key

Recombinant human activated protein C is another drug that acts as an antithrombotic and anti-inflammatory, reducing mortality in patients with sepsis. Alfa Drotrecogin is a human activated protein C that inhibits inflammation, coagulation and improves fibrinolysis. It is contraindicated in patients with active internal bleeding, or who have recently undergone skull surgery and trauma.

Any abscess should be drained. If possible, urinary catheters are removed and possible routes of infection are eliminated (for example, timely replacement of venous catheters). In septic shock, active nutrition of the patient is essential because malnutrition reduces the patient's resistance to infection. Complementary feeding should be started within the first 24 hours of shock (intestinal feeding is preferable to TPN feeding). Continuous infusion of insulin should also be performed to control hyperglycemia. The nurse should work with other members of the health team to find the location and source of the infection and prepare suitable specimens for culture. The patient's hyperthermia (increase in temperature above 40 ° C) should be controlled with acetaminophen, cooling blankets, or ice packs.

The nurse should control shivering when using cooling blankets or ice packs as shivering increases oxygen consumption. Due to reduced blood flow to the kidneys and liver, serum levels of drugs that are naturally cleared by these organs may rise to toxic levels. Therefore, the nurse should check the serum levels of antibiotics, BUN, Cr, WBC and inform the doctor about the increase in their level.

Distributive Shock

- Vessel abnormality leads to dangerously low blood pressure

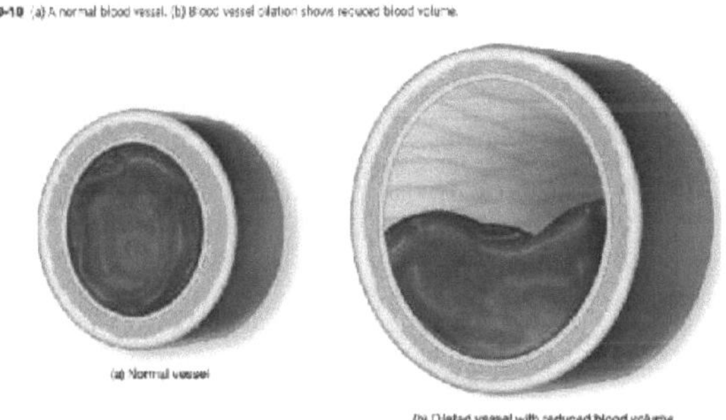

Figure 44. Shock with Annie Colgan Objectives Define shock Describe

Neurogenic shock

This shock may occur following spinal cord injuries, spinal anesthesia, damage to the nervous system, and sometimes a lack of glucose (insulin response) and medications. In neurological shock, vasodilation occurs as a result of an imbalance between sympathetic and parasympathetic stimuli. Sympathetic stimulation causes vascular smooth muscle contraction, and parasympathetic stimulation causes vascular smooth muscle to expand and relax, and the patient experiences a period of vascular relaxation that leads to partial hypovolemia.

Although the volume of blood is sufficient, due to vasodilation, the volume of blood is displaced and a drop in blood pressure occurs. Excessive parasympathetic stimulation causes a decrease in systemic vascular resistance and bradycardia. Insufficient blood pressure causes a lack of tissue and cellular blood flow and causes common conditions in all types of shock. In this shock, the sympathetic system is not able to react to physical stressors and the symptoms of the shock are similar to the manifestations of the sympathetic system. In this shock, unlike other shocks, the skin is hot and dry and the patient has bradycardia.

To prevent shock from spinal anesthesia, the patient's head should be raised 30 degrees to prevent the drug from spreading to the upper parts of the spinal cord. In cases of suspected spinal cord injury, placing the patient in the correct position and keeping the patient immobile can prevent neurogenic shock. Wearing elastic stockings and raising the bottom of the bed, controlling the human symptom and prescribing low molecular weight heparin, and performing inactive range-of-motion movements are some of the ways to prevent and treat venous thrombosis.

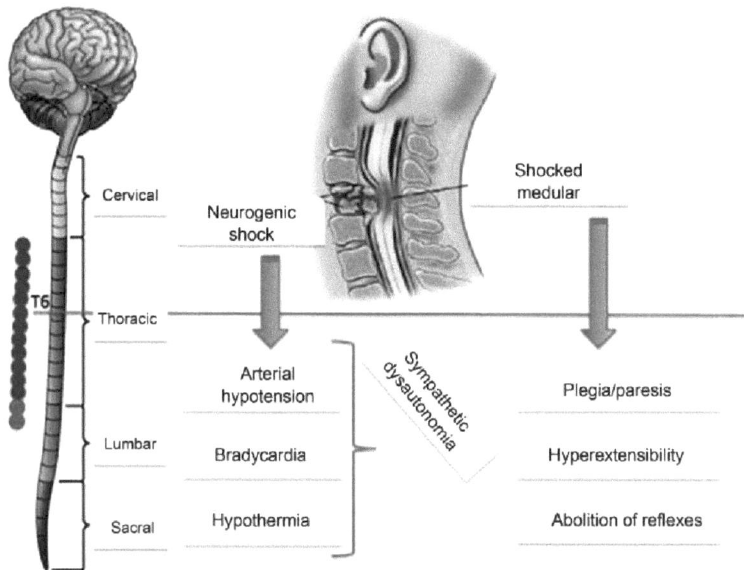

Figure 45. Neurogenic Shock: Clinical Management and Particularities in an Emergency Room

Note: Patients with spinal cord injuries may not report pain from internal injuries, so in the immediate post-injury phase, the patient should be closely monitored for signs of internal bleeding that may cause hypovolemic shock.

Anaphylactic shock: Hypersensitivity to penicillin is the most common cause of anaphylactic shock. This shock occurs due to a general antigen-antibody reaction. To cause such a reaction, the affected patient must be exposed to antigen. This reaction stimulates mast cells and releases substances that affect arteries such as histamine and bradykinin, resulting in diffuse dilation of blood vessels and increased capillary permeability. Treatment includes removal of the causative agents, vascular tone-preserving drugs, and emergency support of vital functions. If cardio-respiratory arrest is possible, CPR should be performed. Epinephrine (vasoconstrictor), diphenhydramine (relieves the effects of histamine and reduces capillary permeability), and albuterol (histamine-induced bronchospasm), including Prescription drugs are anaphylactic shock.

Nursing measures

The main responsibilities of the nurse in relation to shock are to check and recognize the client's condition and to perform the relevant actions and measures in a timely and accurate manner.

The first step in assessing a person with shock is to review the airway, breathing, and circulation quickly and quickly. Then a quick and careful physical examination is performed from head to toe.

Control and improve oxygen delivery: The client should be checked for noisy breathing and airway obstruction. Tracheal deviation (a sign of compressive pneumothorax) should be monitored. In many cases, hypoxia-induced restlessness is confused with pain-induced restlessness, and the person is prescribed narcotic analgesics, which make the condition worse.

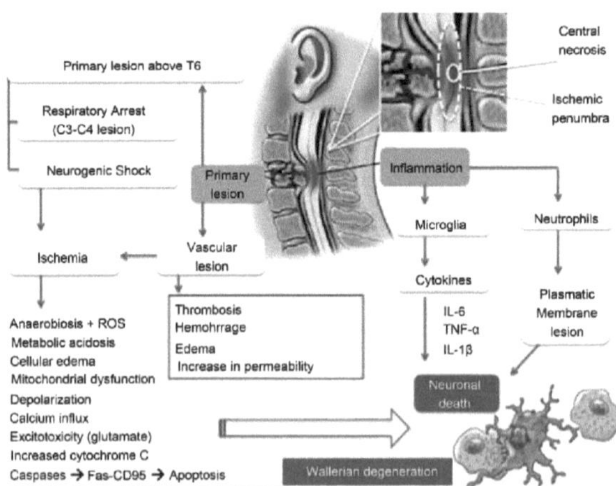

Figure 46. Neurogenic Shock: Clinical Management and Particularities in an Emergency Room

Control of replacement and maintenance of adequate blood flow: pulse, blood pressure, skin color, temperature, peripheral pulses, heart sounds, hydration and blood flow to the skin, condition of mucous membranes, sclera and conjunctiva, paleness or cyanosis of the skin, especially the extremities and peripheral Neck sores should be checked. Despite feeling cold in a shocked client, the heat should not be applied directly to the skin. Local heat causes the peripheral arteries to dilate and blood to be drawn from vital organs to the skin arteries, disrupting the basic compensatory mechanisms of peripheral artery contraction. On the other hand, heat increases metabolism and thus increases the load on the heart to meet the increased need for oxygen. Clients with postural hypotension should not be referred to a radiologist for standing X-rays for complete fluid resuscitation.

Temperature control: Using a flexible anal probe attached to a monitor is an accurate way to control the temperature. The temperature of the tympanic membrane is widely used in vital situations and shows the central temperature of the body. Oral heat control is not only inaccurate but also unsafe.

Cardiac monitoring and hemodynamics: An ECG should be taken to control cardiac activity (although patients are connected to a monitor). During initial resuscitation, care should be taken to place ECG control electrodes on the patient's shoulders, not on the chest. There is no interference with simple chest X-rays, and access to the chest will be better for procedures such as Chest Tube placement, pericardiocentesis, and CPV catheter placement. CVP measurement is necessary to determine the amount of fluid needed to fill the space of the enlarged arteries. Because the CVP only provides preload information, the lines inside the peripheral artery should be fitted with a pulmonary artery catheter sooner. Pulmonary artery pressure and pulmonary capillary wave pressure (PCWP) measurements are also used to assess the left heart and as a guide for fluid administration. Further study and knowledge to prevent further complications are:

- Level of awareness and awareness of the person to time, place and person
- Ability to move limbs

- ➢ Feeling of the limbs
- ➢ The power of grabbing the hands
- ➢ Response to painful or verbal stimuli
- ➢ Pupil size and reaction to light
- ➢ Intestinal sounds, bloating and stiffness in the abdomen, abdominal pain
- ➢ Bad bone shapes
- ➢ Existence of medical warning cards and cards
- ➢ Existence of rupture, crushing, dead blood, petechial and purpura
- ➢ Location, severity, duration of pain and its soothing or aggravating factors

Spinal Shock vs Neurogenic Shock

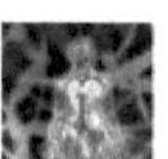

Spinal Shock

- *Due to acute spinal cord injury
- *Absence all voluntary and reflex neurologic activity below level of injury
- Decreased reflexes
- Loss of sensation
- Flaccid paralysis below injury
- Lasts days to months (Transient)
- *Spinal shock & neurogenic shock can in same patient- BUT not same disorder (some sources may group both together)

Neurogenic Shock*

- *Hemodynamic phenomenon-
  - * Loss of vasomotor tone & Loss of sympathetic nervous system tone > inpaired cellular metabolism
- *Critical features-
  - Hypotension (due to massive vasodilation
  - Bradycardia- due to unopposed paraynmpathetic stimulation
  - Poikilothermia; *Unable to regulate temperature-
- Occurs
  - Within 30 min cord injury level T 5 or above; last up to 6 weeks; also due to effect some drugs that effect vasomotor center of medulla as opioids, benzodiazedines
- Management (*Determine underlying cause)
  - Airway support
  - Fluids as needed- Typically 0.9 NS , rate depends upon need
  - Atropine for bradycardia
  - Vasopressors as phenylelphrine (Neo-synephrine) for BP support

Figure 47. Pin on Nursing Skills

Chapter VI

Cardiogenic Shock in ICU

Cardiogenic shock may be due to arrhythmia, myocardial infarction due to ischemia, systemic or pulmonary hypertension, myocarditis, or myocardiopathy. Diagnosis is usually based on a known history of cardiovascular disease with an abnormal ECG in a patient in shock with dilated cervical veins.

Prognosis: In the treatment of this disease, it is necessary to strike a balance between improving cardiac output and reducing oxygen demand and myocardial workload. This balance must be achieved while maintaining heart muscle perfusion. The prognosis of cardiogenic shock depends on finding and resolving the underlying cause. Cardiogenic shock requires immediate action, often before the underlying cause is identified.

Diagnostic signs and symptoms

♦ Hypotension due to decreased blood flow to less than normal blood flow.

♦ Tachycardia due to the heart trying to pump blood faster to maintain adequate blood flow to the body, or sometimes bradycardia due to myocardial injury where the heart rate is less than 60 beats per minute.

♦ Arrhythmias - When the heart muscle does not receive enough oxygen, it becomes irritable, resulting in arrhythmias.

♦ Cold and moist skin due to reduced tissue oxygenation.

♦ Decreased skin temperature due to decreased blood flow as a result of hypotension.

♦ Decreased urinary output to less than 30 ml / h (oliguria) due to decreased renal blood flow.

♦ Secondary pulmonary tingling sound to pulmonary edema due to accumulation of fluid in the lungs.

♦ Confusion due to insufficient cerebral perfusion.

♦ Dilation of the jugular veins due to the heart's inability to manage blood flow back to the heart, which is a sign of fluid overload.

♦ Bruising of the lips and limbs as a result of poor blood circulation.

Slow heart rate (less than 50 beats per minute) can cause inadequate heart output; Because cardiac output is the product of the volume of beats and the number of heartbeats. The rapid heartbeat - which is too much to subtract 230 from the patient's age by year - can lead to inadequate cardiac output due to the short time it takes for the ventricles to fill and the coronary arteries to bleed during diastole.

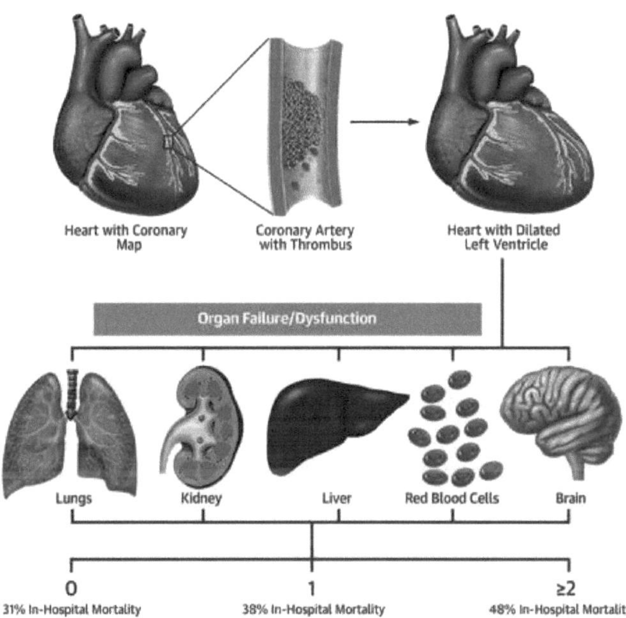

Figure 48. Acute Noncardiac Organ Failure in Acute Myocardial Infarction With Cardiogenic Shock

Myocardial ischemia due to insufficient oxygen; Anatomical defects due to ineffective contraction; Hypertension due to increased ventricular load and disorders caused by dilation or hypertrophy of the myocardium; And myocardial infarction can cause shock due to internal heart muscle failure.

The diagnosis of cardiogenic shock usually depends on the diagnosis of the underlying disease. Shock, dilated cervical veins, peripheral edema, large and sensitive liver, third heart sound, ischemic symptoms on ECG, and enlarged heart on chest x-ray can help with the diagnosis. Diagnosis is usually simple, but in two common cases it can be difficult. The first is a ruptured abdominal aortic aneurysm in a patient with coronary artery disease. The diagnostic key is examination of the cervical veins. The second condition is shock due to myocardial infarction in a patient with a major chest injury. Blunt trauma to the chest can cause heart damage, but such damage usually leads to immediate death.

Treatment: Narcotic analgesics, which are especially effective in treating heart failure following myocardial infarction.

Diuretics: Diuretics are an ideal treatment for congestive heart failure with increased vascular volume, but are used in cardiovascular disorders caused by hypovolemia, trauma, compression of the heart, sepsis, or loss of microvascular tone.

Chronotropic drugs: Patients with heart failure with bradycardia may rarely and temporarily benefit from chronotropic drugs such as atropine or isoproterenol.

Inotropic drugs: Low doses of these drugs increase myocardial contractility. In addition, dopamine appears to dilate renal arteries, increasing renal blood flow and urinary output. The main use of these drugs is to increase blood flow in the cardiovascular system; Dopamine, unlike dobotamine, typically dramatically increases heart rate. Dopamine and dobutamine should be used with caution and the patient should be monitored in the ICU. These drugs cause systemic arterioles to contract at doses of 10 μg / kg / min or more. Even low doses in hypovolemic patients (for example, 5μg / kg / min dopamine) can cause ischemic necrosis of the fingers.

Vasodilators: The most useful vasodilators in surgical patients with heart failure are morphine sulfate, nitroprusside, and nitroglycerin, all of which are easily reversible or short-acting.

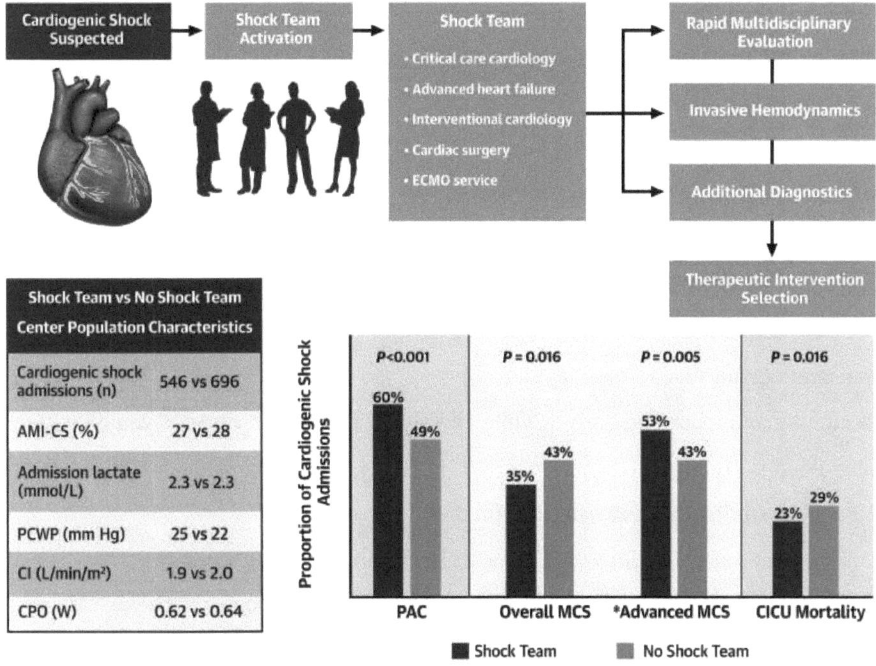

Figure 49. Management and Outcomes of Cardiogenic Shock in Cardiac ICUs With Versus Without Shock

Nursing interventions

♦Monitor vital signs - check for changes in blood pressure, pulse, respiration.

♦ Monitor heart sounds

♦ Swanz Ganz Catheter Monitor - A catheter that is inserted into a pulmonary artery to check for cardiovascular and pulmonary pressure.

♦ Capillary filling test.

♦ Monitor arterial blood gas to test pH, acidosis or alkalosis, bicarbonate level.

♦ Respiratory monitoring - Due to poor perfusion, these patients develop respiratory distress, mechanical ventilation may be required.

♦ Putting the patient to absolute rest.

♦ Monitoring fluid intake and excretion (I / O) - Check adequate renal perfusion. Without effective cardiac function, the patient will not have enough renal blood flow for adequate blood filtration.

♦ Teach the patient the following:

♦ Signs and symptoms that you should take care of and inform your doctor or nurse if it occurs.

♦ Rest intervals between activities.

♦ Contact a nurse or doctor if you notice weight gain, shortness of breath, fatigue, dependent edema.

♦ Weighing and recording daily weight, contacting a doctor or nurse if you gain more than 3 pounds (1.4 kg).

♦ Change your diet to a low-salt, low-fat diet.

Definitions of SCAI Shock Stages WITH CICU, Hospital Mortality

CENTRAL ILLUSTRATION: Definitions of SCAI Shock Stages A Through E, With Associated Cardiac Intensive Care Unit and Hospital Mortality in Each SCAI Shock Stage

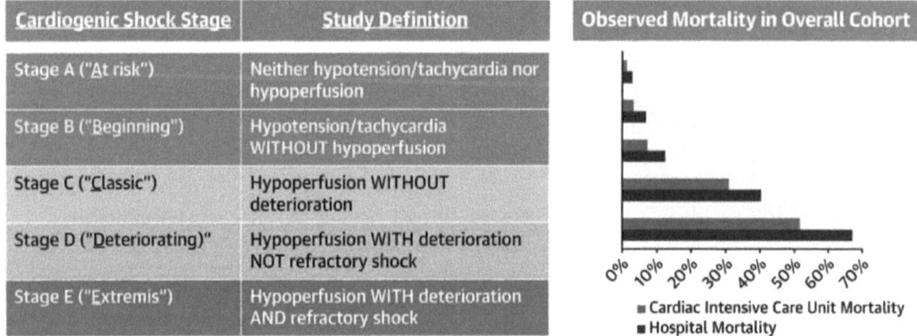

Cardiogenic Shock Stage	Study Definition
Stage A ("At risk")	Neither hypotension/tachycardia nor hypoperfusion
Stage B ("Beginning")	Hypotension/tachycardia WITHOUT hypoperfusion
Stage C ("Classic")	Hypoperfusion WITHOUT deterioration
Stage D ("Deteriorating)"	Hypoperfusion WITH deterioration NOT refractory shock
Stage E ("Extremis")	Hypoperfusion WITH deterioration AND refractory shock

Figure 50. An Update on Acute Mechanical Circulatory Support in Cardiogenic Shock

Chapter VII

Shock Emergency in ICU

General pre-hospital measures for dealing with shock victims

1- Observe BSI precautions.

In trauma patients, even wear latex gloves where possible due to the possibility of contact with blood and other secretions. Wear protective goggles if necessary, especially when injured.

2- Evaluate the scene size (scene size up). In the stage evaluation stage, pay attention to the following:

A) Make sure the safety and security of the scene.

Your safety and that of your co-worker should not be compromised during the mission. You need to make sure there is no risk of explosion or re-accident and other risk factors at the scene. These conditions are usually achieved with the presence of relief agents such as police, fire brigade, etc.

B) Investigate the mechanism of injury leading to shock.

Like other types of traumata, familiarity with the mechanism of injury plays an important role in the suspicion of injuries to organs leading to shock, such as the abdomen, pelvis, chest, spine, etc. Penetrating and blunt (non-penetrating) trauma can lead to damage to these organs.

C) Make sure you have sufficient resources and facilities at your disposal.

If you have a high probability of a casualty and failure to provide services to them or the possibility of needing other rescue agents to release the injured, request an additional ambulance or other rescue agents.

Note: In case of access to the casualty, for the initial assessment, maintain the stability of the spine and give the casualty a suitable position.

3- Carry out the primary assessment of the casualty based on the priority of ABCDE measures

A) Determine the stimulus response status (level of consciousness) of the casualty based on the AVPU and GCS criteria. Decreased or non-response of the casualty to stimuli (loss of consciousness) indicates the potential for a life-threatening problem that helps diagnose the casualty's emergency and critical condition.

B) Evaluate and maintain the initial assessment of the casualty based on ABCDE. Evaluate the casualty's airway for openness, and in case of any airway obstruction, take action to open it: Airway. The open airway (free and clean) proves by talking (speaking) the casualty normally for a few seconds and the absence of abnormal sound, in which case you should go to the assessment of breathing or Breathing. Airway obstruction may manifest as abnormal sounds in the upper airway, such as snoring, grunting, stridor or agitation, and eventually respiratory distress due to the inability to speak or speak. In this case, you must first open the airway with appropriate techniques and then proceed to maintain and maintain it with the following measures.

I. To open the airway in the injured with a reduced level of consciousness; Use jaw thrust or chin lift maneuvers.
II. Removal of secretions and other substances in the airway:
III. If there is blood and secretions, you should suction and if there are other cases such as foreign objects, remove it with a sweeping finger. If the denture is obstructed, remove it, otherwise fix it in place.
IV. After opening the airway, you must maintain the open airway. Auxiliary devices such as oral-pharyngeal airway (OPA), nasopharyngeal airway (NPA) can be used to keep the airway open if needed. If these measures fail to open or close the airway, advanced airway management such as endotracheal intubation (ETT), laryngeal mask (LMA) may be unavoidable.

Note: In assessing the condition of the injured airway; Decreased level of consciousness, inability to speak (speech), the presence of abnormal sounds in the upper airway and the presence of respiratory distress indicate a critical or critical condition in the casualty that the necessary measures should be taken.

Collar-C: In spinal cord injury, especially those who are fully conscious but have symptoms of vertebral injury, as well as all casualties who have altered levels of consciousness, consider immobilizing the spine. First, completely immobilize the head and neck with your hands. Then fix the cervical vertebrae with the neck clarinet and continue to immobilize the head and neck with the hand until the dorsal spine is fixed using a long backboard and fixed with an immobilizer head or pad.

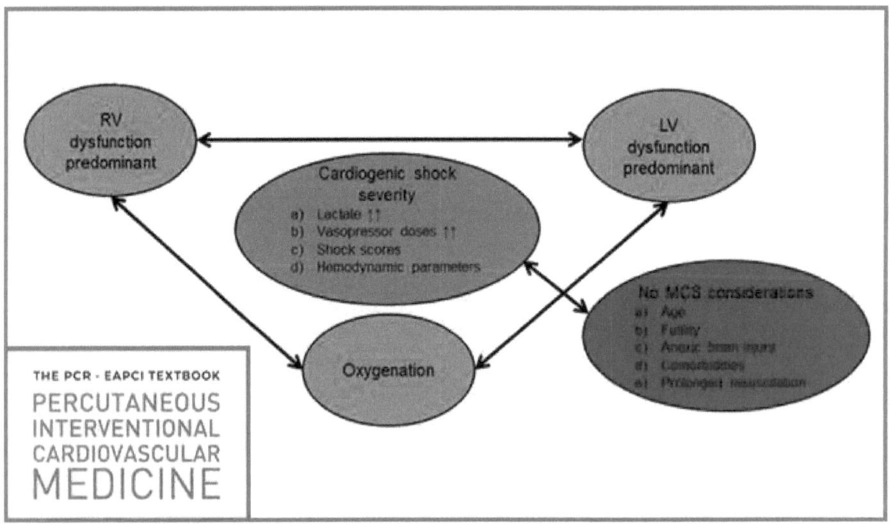

Figure 51. All you need to know on cardiogenic shock

Breathing: Assess and maintain the patient's breathing status. In general, after ensuring that the airway is open, take the following steps to maintain and assess the casualty's respiratory status:

A) View the chest (LOOK)

The following should be considered when viewing an injured chest:

- **Chest ups and downs:** If the injured chest does not go up and down and the patient does not have breathing (respiratory apnea), auxiliary ventilation should be established immediately using an oxygen-sealed bag (BMV) mask attached to the oxygen and then continue the evaluation. Also check the injured chest for penetrating and sucking wounds, bruising, contradictory movements, tracheal deviation, bulging jugular veins, etc.
- **Number of casualties:** Anaerobic metabolism due to decreased cellular oxygenation increases lactic acid production. Hydrogen ions from acidosis and hypoxia stimulate the respiratory center and increase the number and depth of ventilation. Therefore, tachypnea is usually considered one of the first signs of shock. The number of casualties per minute (adults, children, and infants) should be determined. In patients with shock, if breathing is slow (less than 12 breaths per minute) or rapid or tachypnea (20-30 breaths per minute) or very rapid (more than 30 breaths per minute) First, auxiliary oxygen is administered by an oxygen mask, and if not corrected, ventilation should be started immediately using BMV.
- **Injured breathing depth:** In assessing the casualty's respiratory status, the depth of breathing should be evaluated to determine if the patient's breathing depth is normal or if the breathing is shallow. If there is shallow breathing, auxiliary oxygen should first be administered with an oxygen mask, and if not corrected, ventilation using BMV should be started immediately.

B) Listen to the chest (Listen)

Lung hearing should be done by a medical phone in terms of the presence of normal and equal or unequal breathing sounds (Unequal-Equal) and also the presence of abnormal breathing sounds such as whistling, etc. Injuries that interfere with the ventilation process and reduce respiratory sounds in the lungs include pneumothorax, compression pneumothorax, hemothrax, and lung contusion.

C) Touch the chest (Fell)

If the casualty is ventilated, you should immediately expose, monitor, and touch the casualty chest. In touching the chest, one should pay attention to conditions such as tenderness, cryptos, etc.

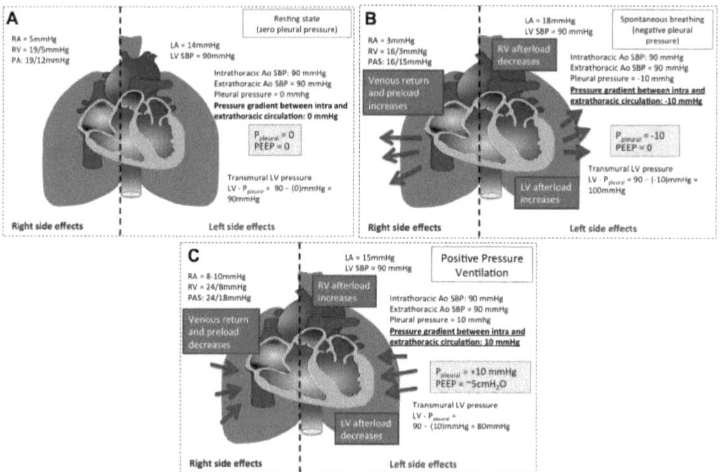

Figure 52. Positive Pressure Ventilation in Cardiogenic Shock

D) Supply of supplementary and additional oxygen

In all shock patients, especially if the casualty is disturbed in ventilation and distress, start with a simple oxygen mask at 8 to 10 liters per minute and a 15-liter oxygen reserve mask per minute, regardless of the amount of oxygen saturation. It is necessary to use auxiliary and excess oxygen to the extent that the concentration reaches 85% or more, in such injuries, at least until their general condition is immobilized. In general, you should not trust the ability of this group of injured people to provide the oxygen they need and always watch over them in view of the deteriorating general condition. If the casualty is breathing (Brady Penne), rapid breathing (Taki Penne), shallow and ineffective breathing, and does not improve with the use of mask oxygenation and the concentration or FIO_2 does not reach 85%, ventilation should be used.

Note: When giving assisted breathing (especially to an injured person with hypovolemic shock) care should be taken not to experience hyperventilation. Very deep and fast ventilation causes alkalosis in the injured person. Alkalosis also shifts the oxyhemoglobin curve to the right, thereby increasing the hemoglobin's affinity for oxygen. As a result, oxygen transport to the tissues is reduced.

Note: In assessing the injured breathing condition (Breathing); Lack of chest ups and downs, number of rapid and slow breaths, shallow breathing, reduction or absence of breathing sounds, cyanosis, tenderness, cryptography, emphysema, suction wound, tracheal deviation, jugular vein bulge, indicating critical condition or critical (critical) in the injured that necessary measures should be taken.

Circulation: Assessing and maintaining blood circulation. After assessing the casualty's respiratory status and ensuring respiratory adequacy, assessing the presence or disturbance of the circulatory system is the next step in caring for a spinal cord injury victim. At initial evaluation, external bleeding should be identified and controlled immediately. After this, they can: a) general circulatory status and adequacy of tissue perfusion, b) radial pulse assessment, c) skin color assessment, d) temperature assessment, and) skin moisture, and e) capillary filling time. Also, measures such as intravenous implantation and serum therapy are performed if the patient's condition is unstable.

A) Control of external bleeding

Detect any external bleeding immediately and control it with direct pressure (Direct pressure and tourniquet). If internal bleeding is suspected, the injured abdomen should be examined immediately for signs of injury. Examine the femurs as well: Fractures of the pelvis and femurs are an important source of internal bleeding. Injured, as well as rapid replacement of hot intravenous fluid care.

Note: however, that many causes of bleeding cannot be easily controlled outside the hospital. Prehospital care in these cases is the immediate transfer of the injured to a trauma center equipped with facilities and personnel to control bleeding immediately in the operating room.

B) Radial pulse assessment

First touch the radial pulse of the casualty. If the radial pulse in an upper limb is not palpable without injury, the casualty may have entered a non-compensatory phase of shock, which is a sign of deterioration.

If the casualty does not have a radial pulse, touch the carotid pulse. If the carotid and femoral pulse is not palpable in the casualty, it is because he has heart or lung disease.

If the casualty had a radial pulse, evaluate the pulse for the following:

Rate: Determine if the casualty's pulse rate is fast / normal / slow. The presence of a rapid pulse in trauma patients will cause the loss of blood volume due to internal and external bleeding and the possibility of hemorrhagic and neurogenic shock. Existence of slow pulse Evidence of pulse strength (Volume): Determine whether the injured pulse strength is strong / weak. Poor pulse in trauma patients is the reason for the loss of blood volume due to internal and external bleeding and the possibility of hemorrhagic and neurogenic shock. Pulse also provides information about systolic blood pressure.

C) Skin color assessment: Evaluate the injured skin color. The presence of pink skin color is the reason for good tissue perfusion. Pale skin indicates a decrease in tissue perfusion and the cause of hemorrhage. Bruising of the skin is the reason for insufficient oxygen supply.

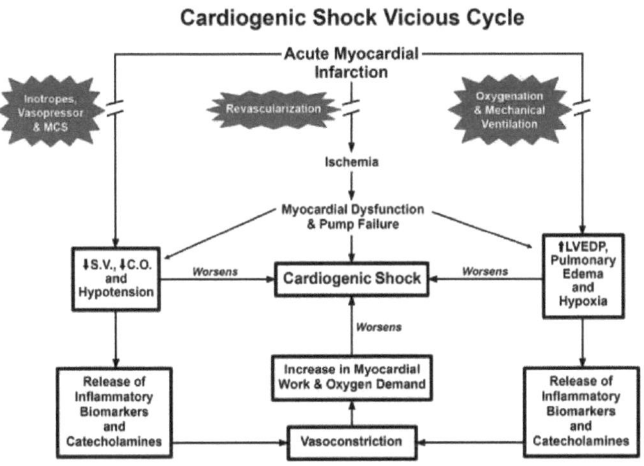

Figure 53. Cardiogenic Shock

D) Skin temperature assessment: Assess the injured skin temperature. Cold skin indicates a decrease in perfusion, for whatever reason. When wearing gloves, the temperature of the skin should be determined by touching the back of the hand.

F) Evaluate skin moisture: Assess the moisture of the injured skin Dry skin is the reason for good perfusion. Wet skin indicates shock and reduced perfusion.

E) Evaluation of capillary refill time: If this time is more than 2 seconds, the reason is that capillary substrates do not receive sufficient perfusion.

Note: In assessing the condition of the injured circulation (Circulation); External bleeding, possibility of internal bleeding, rapid radial pulse, slow and weak pulse, pale skin and bruised or cyanotic skin, cold and wet skin, as well as re-reduction of tissue filling, indicating critical or severe condition (Critical) In the injured that the necessary measures should be taken.

Fixing and transferring the injured to the ambulance

After correcting airway obstruction and oxygen delivery to the lungs, as well as controlling external bleeding, fix the casualty with a long, spider-shaped backboard and transport him to the ambulance. In case of suspected spinal cord injury, this should be done more carefully and sensitively, and the casualty should be fixed and transferred to the backboard in a fully integrated manner.

Prepare the patient to be sent to the medical center.

In patients with abdominal and pelvic trauma, especially critically injured, do the Circulation at the scene until the end of the Circulation phase, and then immediately transfer the patient to the medical center to continue the work and the next steps. And continue to work and take action along the way.

Disability: Assessing the neurological status.

Assessment of brain function through assessment of level of consciousness (GCS), pupil assessment, and sensory and motor assessment in all trauma victims is considered part of routine assessment after circulatory assessment. This assessment plays a very important role in the care, transmission and triage of spinal cord injury patients. At this point in assessing the casualty, do the following:

A) Assess the level of consciousness: Determine the level of consciousness of the casualty based on the AVPU or GCS criteria. Decreased or non-response of the casualty to stimuli (loss of consciousness) indicates the potential for a life-threatening problem that helps diagnose the casualty's emergency and critical condition. Decreased level of consciousness (LOC) also considered the aggressive and aggressive casualty to be hypoxia-injured until proven otherwise.

B) Assess the condition of the pupils: Examine the injured pupils for size and reflex response to light and symmetry. The presence of unequal pupils in an anesthetized trauma casualty may be a reason for the pressure on the third cerebral nerve (responsible for the contraction and dilation of the pupils) due to increased intracranial (ICP) following edema of the brain or an expanding intracranial hematoma. Because in this case, with increasing intracranial pressure, pressure is applied to the brainstem (Brain Stem) and causes pressure on the third cranial nerve.

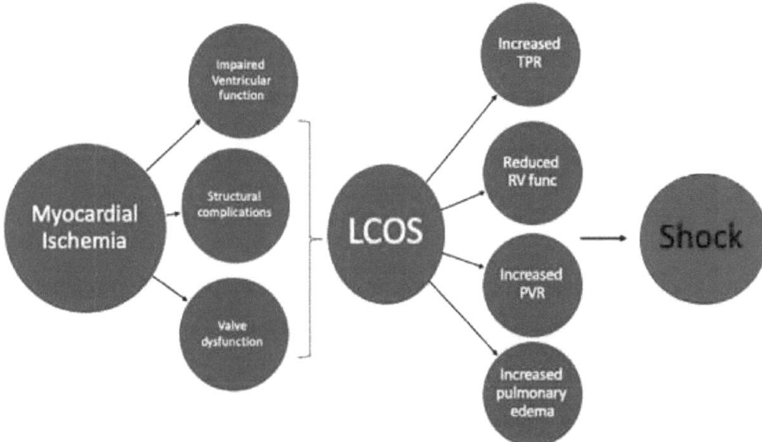

Figure 54. Coronary Artery Bypass Grafting in Cardiogenic Shock: Decision-Making, Management Options

C) Evaluation of sensation and movement of limbs: At this stage, based on diagnostic tests to assess sensation and movement, the damaged areas in the CNS can be identified and these areas that need further examination can be taken care of.

Exposure: Assessing hidden damage / external environment. At this stage, the hidden injuries of the injured are evaluated. Injured people with spinal cord trauma can also suffer from other injuries that may be life-threatening. Therefore, their whole body needs to be examined for potentially fatal injuries. This step includes the following steps:

A) Undress the patient: By maintaining the privacy of the injured and observing ethical points, by exposing the injured, if necessary, investigate the hidden life-threatening injuries in the injured with chest trauma.

B) Prevention of hypothermia: In trauma casualties, especially after stripping the casualty, hypothermia is considered a serious problem in the process of caring for trauma casualties. Only the part that is needed should be in contact with the outside environment. When the complete examination of the casualty is completed inside the EMS hot unit, it is necessary to cover him again immediately to prevent hypothermia.

3) Preventing Hypothermia Injured: In pre-hospital conditions, after hypothermia occurs, raising the core body temperature is a problem, so all necessary measures to maintain body temperature should be taken at the scene of the accident. The following measures should be taken to prevent hypothermia:

- Any wet clothes, including clothes soaked in blood, should be removed from the injured body, because wet clothes cause more waste of body heat.
- The injured body should be covered with warm blankets. Or you can use plastic sheets. These sheets are disposable and inexpensive, easy to maintain and are effective tools for maintaining body temperature.
- If it is possible to use hot and humid oxygen, it can help maintain body temperature, especially in intubated casualties.
- Transfer the injured to a warm ambulance cabin. Keep the ambulance temperature at 29 ° C for severely injured people. The rate of heat dissipation of an injured person in a cold place is very high. Conditions for the injured, not the technicians, should be ideal, because in any emergency situation, the most important person is the injured.

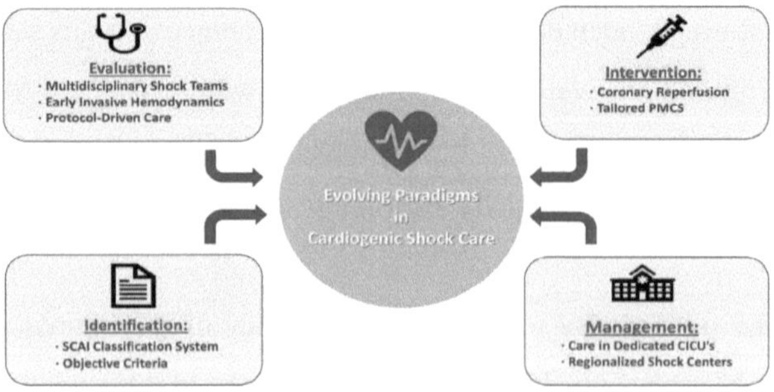

Figure 55. Aging, Evolving paradigms in cardiogenic shock care

4) Rapid transfer to a suitable medical center: Two urgent needs of the injured with severe hemorrhagic shock are: blood transfusion and also a surgeon with access to the operating room. Because neither of these two conditions is routinely present in the pre-hospital, the rapid transfer of the casualty to a medical facility that has facilities to care for the casualty is extremely important. Rapid transfer does not mean neglecting important care measures for the casualty, but technicians must immediately take basic and rescue measures, such as opening the airway, restoring breathing, and controlling bleeding. Inappropriate assessment methods and unnecessary immobilization maneuvers should not be wasted time. When a critically ill casualty is to be cared for, many care measures, such as warming the casualty, taking a blood vessel, and even a secondary evaluation, can be performed in an ambulance while the casualty is being transported.

Use of shock-proof pants (PASG): Use of shock-proof pants or PASG can be temporarily helpful in dealing with severe hemorrhagic shock. This device increases vascular resistance and reduces the volume of the vessel, and at the same time causes tamponade of abdominal and pelvic bleeding. The most important use of PASG is to control intra-abdominal and pelvic bleeding in people with blood pressure below 60 mm Hg. However, because PASG raises the casualty's blood pressure, bleeding from areas outside the device increases.

C) Examination and complete observation of suspicious parts of the injured body.
In an acceptable initial assessment, all dangerous injuries should be identified and the necessary measures should be taken to cause secondary complications in them. To achieve this important goal, all parts of the body must be evaluated and clinically examined.

- Chest
- Belly
- The pelvis
- Organs

D) Logroll the injured to check the back.

The back area should be evaluated for any latent or fatal injuries. Of course, this can be done when rolling the casualty to place a long backboard.

5) Transfer of the injured.

In order to achieve the best possible result, it is necessary to transfer the injured with abdominal and pelvic trauma directly to the trauma center, which is equipped with facilities and immediate surgery. If such a center is not available, air transfer from the scene of the accident to a suitable center can be considered.

6) Perform a secondary assessment of the patient.

After the initial evaluation of the patient, in order to identify and treat life-threatening conditions that affect the level of consciousness, airway, respiration and circulation, the next step is to perform a secondary evaluation followed by other care and treatment measures. Of course, the place and time of doing so depends on the decision to make an immediate transfer or to continue the actions on the scene. The patient's secondary assessment includes reviewing and performing the following:

A) Obtain a SAMPLE-based re-history: Obtain a re-history of the patient from the patient himself, his companion, or witnesses at the scene, and ask about SAMPLE components.

B) Control of the patient's vital signs.

Monitor and record vital signs of injury including PR, BP, RR, SPO2 and even BS if needed.

C) Performing thorough examinations from head to toe.

Perform a thorough head-to-toe examination at this stage again. So that no abnormal points are hidden from your view.

7) Carry out continuous evaluation and continuation of medical care and support of the injured during sending to the medical center

Intravenous implantation: Use a large angiocatheter (green, gray, or brick) to secure the patient with one or two intravenous routes for drug or serum injections.

Replacement of lost fluids: Dehydrated casualties need to be replaced with fluids and salt, while trauma casualties who have lost blood require blood replacement. Because blood transfusions are not available in pre-hospital settings, an intravenous electrolyte solution should be injected into trauma patients with bleeding. The best solutions to replace lost body fluids are crystalloid solutions. In the treatment of hemorrhagic shock, lactated Ringer's solution is the best alternative to blood.

Normal saline crystalloid solution can also be used to replace the lost volume, but may cause hyperchloremia (increased blood chloride concentration) and eventually acidosis. If there are signs of shock, the infusion of fluids is done first at a rate of 1 liter, then the clinical signs of the casualty are evaluated, if the symptoms of shock were somewhat resolved (especially radial pulse touch or BP> 9), the infusion of fluids is stopped. But if the symptoms of foot shock are still present, another 1 liter of fluid is infused again. Check blood glucose levels for casualties with abnormal GCS scores. If hypoglycemia is present, 50% dextrose solution can be injected to return blood sugar to normal.

CBR and relaxation of the patient: Restless patients should have CBR at the earliest opportunity because the more physical activity the patient has, the greater the respiratory activity and the greater the need for oxygen. Also reduce the patient's anxiety and fear. Reassure the patient.

Patient position: For injured people with spinal trauma, supine position is the most appropriate and stable position and it is necessary to try to keep the injured person in this position when moving and moving.

- Relieve the pain of the injured: If possible, to relieve the pain of the injured, prescribe painkillers.
- During dispatch, you should check the following items every 5 minutes:

➢ Level of consciousness of the injured: About 3% of the injured with mild brain damage (GCS = 14-15) may have an unforeseen disturbance of consciousness. Injuries that lose more than 2 GCS points during the transfer are at risk of injury. These injured need to be transported quickly to a suitable medical center. This change in consciousness should also be reported to the recipient medical center.

Injured responses to care and treatment measures should also be reported.

- Respiratory status in terms of increase, decrease and irregularity of its rate.
- Pulse status in terms of the number of decreases.
- Blood pressure status in terms of increased systolic pressure and flattened pulse pressure.
- If the level of consciousness of the pupils decreases in terms of dilation and reaction to light.

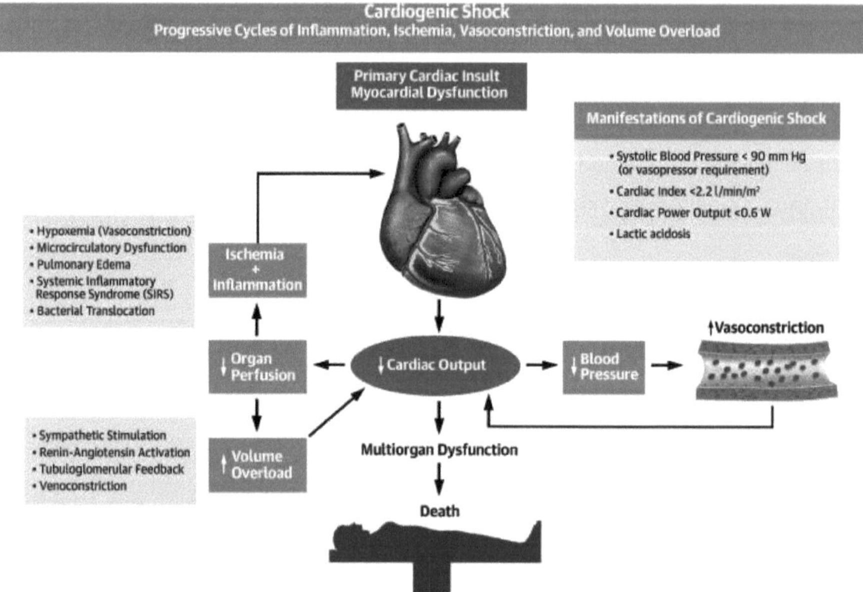

Figure 56. A Standardized and Comprehensive Approach to the Management of Cardiogenic Shock

8) Communication with destination medical centers.

During direct contact with the destination medical center or via dispatch, the receiving center should be notified as soon as possible so that they can make the necessary preparations by the time the casualty arrives. This communication and reporting can be done by radio (wireless) or by telephone and should include the mechanism of the accident, GCS and early vital signs, any change in posture during transmission, the presence of local signs (such as motor asymmetry, Unilateral or bilateral dilatation of the pupils), other serious injuries, and casualty response to primary care measures.

9) Documentation

While documenting all findings on the mission sheet in writing, you should contact the destination emergency directly or via dispatch and provide a summary of the patient's condition to the destination (orally).

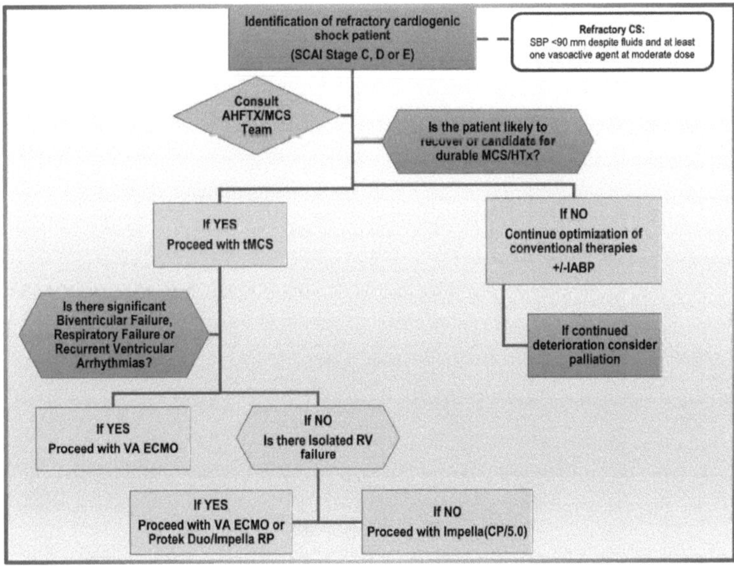

Figure 57. Mechanical Circulatory Support in Cardiogenic Shock: Shock Team or Bust?

Chapter VIII

Nursing and Shock

Shock is a factor or factors that endanger human life and is divided into the following types:

1- Loss of body fluids.

2- Distributed shock which includes: infectious-neurological-psychological and allergic.

3- Heart.

Loss of body fluids: This type of shock occurs in two ways, which is caused by heavy bleeding and late arrival of fluids to the body. If an injured person bleeds internally or externally for a variety of reasons and we cannot control it immediately after the accident, he or she will experience a shock of dehydration. Symptoms of this shock can include restlessness, anxiety, and shortness of breath. Some limbs are cold sweat thirsty and later accompanied by anesthesia.

Cardiogenic shock

First aid for these people

First we do the initial evaluation, which included ABCH. Keep the person warm. Put the person in recovery mode or raise the patient's foot about 30 cm above the ground and take the person to a medical center if this loss of body fluids through diarrhea is the most common cause of death in children. If done, we must use ORS powders and take the injured to medical centers.

Distributed shock: Infectious shock, which is one of the most common causes of death, is caused by a virus entering the body, which causes a person to have a fever, high blood pressure, and high heart rate.

We perform the necessary first aid assessment, including the ABC, and identify the cause of the shock and take the person to a medical center.

Nerve shock: Any factor in the human nervous system and nervous system, such as falling from heights or rocks and getting hit in the spine, causes this shock. Symptoms include no organ reaction and no urinary or fecal stimulation.

First Aid: We perform the initial evaluation including ABC and transfer the injured to medical centers while maintaining the spinal problem.

Psychological shock: Psychological shock or fainting that can be caused by hearing an unfortunate incident or seeing heartbreaking scenes.

Symptoms: Seeing light spots (black and dark eyes) Dizziness - Anesthesia.

First aid: First, we protect the person from falling so that he does not get broken, then we raise him 20 to 30 cm below his feet, let the oxygen reach the person easily and do not crowd around him. After full consciousness, we can give him fluids or sugar water. This anesthesia may take 4 or 5 minutes. If it is more than this time, we will definitely perform the initial evaluation measures and transfer him to the medical centers.

Do not: We do not slap the injured person until we give him full consciousness of liquids, we do not spray water on his face.

Severe allergic shock: This type of shock, which is mild and severe and can be dangerous to the human body, requires special first aid. This type of shock can be caused by insect bites, food additives or certain medications. Basically, this type of shock causes premature death due to a disorder of the respiratory system. Symptoms include cough, shortness of breath, swelling of the face and tongue, dizziness, unconsciousness, severe itching, nausea and vomiting.

First Aid: Solve ABC initial assessment and respiratory problems. We use drugs such as bipolar or epinephrine. Heart attack is one of the most common circulatory system problems and can be treated briefly and simply.

Comparison of different types of shock

Hypovolemic	Hypotension, tachycardia Weak thready pulse Cool, pale, moist skin U/O decreased	Decreased CO **Increased SVR**
Cardiogenic	Hypotension, tachycardia Weak thready pulse Cool, pale, moist skin U/O < 30 ml/hr Crackles, tachypnea	Decreased CO Increased SVR
Neurogenic	Hypotension, BRADYCARDIA **WARM DRY SKIN**	Decreased CO **Venous & arterial vasodilation, loss sympathetic tone**
Anaphylactic	Hypotension, tachycardia Cough, dyspnea Pruritus, urticaria Restlessness, decreased LOC	Decreased CO Decreased SVR
Septic	Hypotension, Tachycardia Full bounding pulse, tachypnea **Pink, warm, flushed skin** Decreased U/O, fever	**Decreased** CO, **Decreased** SVR

Figure 58. Types of Shock Cheat Sheet, Nursing school survival, ICU nursing, Nursing school notes

Hypertension: The symptoms of this complication are due to clogged arteries or a virus entering the body and its symptoms are headache and dizziness. Pain sensation for more than 2 minutes in the heart and left hand.

We put the first aid person in a sitting position so that the angle of the head decreases from 90 degrees, and then if the pressure is higher than 160, we give him sublingual nitroglycerin for 20 minutes. We check his pressure and if he does not come down again, we will use this method. For the third time, we will definitely move to the medical center and treat the person there.

Low blood pressure: Symptoms of dizziness, weakness and darkening of the eyes.

First Aid: Preventing a person from falling. Raising the soles of the feet between 20 and 30 cm.

Note: The use of some of the mentioned drugs must be done with the order of a doctor or a qualified person, otherwise the helper is not allowed.

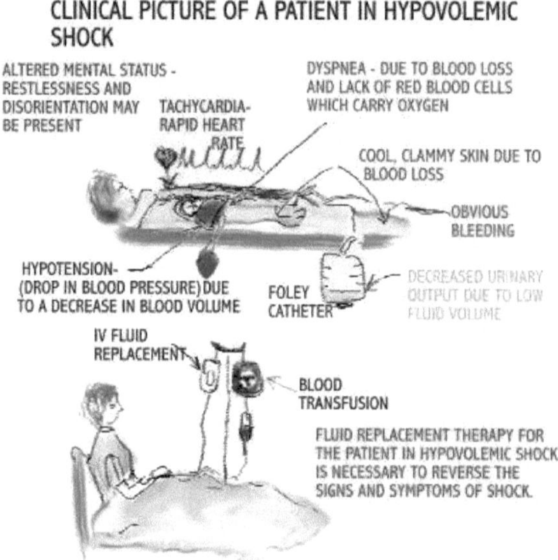

Figure 59. Dear Nurses: ICU nursing, Nursing school survival, Critical care nursing

Body reaction to shock

Decreased blood flow to vital organs such as the heart and brain can cause irreversible damage within minutes. To prevent such damage, the body activates a series of compensatory mechanisms to establish a steady flow of blood to the brain and heart, which reduces blood flow to less important and insensitive organs such as the skin and muscles. The first stage) and in the next stages, the kidneys and other abdominal organs and intestines are done. At the same time, the heart rate increases to help increase blood flow to the vascular system. These compensatory mechanisms are affected by the sympathetic nervous system and adrenal hormones (epinephrine and pyenephrine tape). The body's reaction to insufficient blood supply to the tissues and organs of the body (shock) causes the initial symptoms of shock.

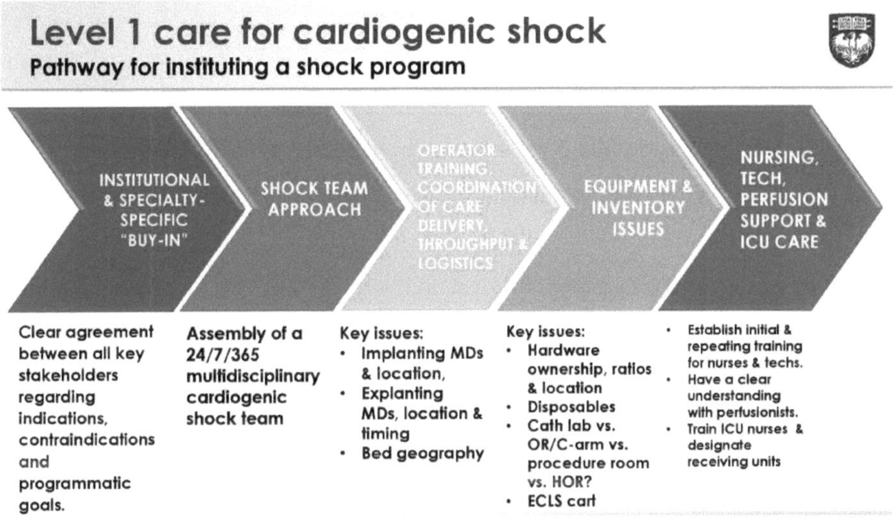

Figure 60. Key elements of a cardiogenic shock team

Causes of shock

The heart and blood vessels form the vascular reservoir in the human body that holds blood, and normal blood flow is affected by three factors: the heart's contractile strength, blood volume, and blood vessel diameter. If any of these three pressure factors; Cardiac pumping, blood volume, and dilation and contraction of blood vessels are impaired and do not function properly, blood supply to body tissues will not be adequate and shock will occur. Hence, shock can be divided into three general types.

Shock caused by decreased blood volume.

Shock caused by decreased heart strength.

Shock caused by dilation of blood vessels.

Shock caused by decreased blood volume.

Shock due to fluid loss for any reason is called volume shock or hypovolemic shock. The most common type of shock that is also dangerous in the injured is hypovolemic shock or shock due to decreased blood volume. Decreased blood volume can be directly due to blood loss (for example, in external and internal bleeding) or plasma (for example, in extensive burns, etc.). In most cases, volume shock is due to bleeding, which is called bleeding shock or hemorrhagic shock.

It should be emphasized that blood is only a small part of all body fluids. All body fluids together make up about 60% of the total body weight. Decreased blood plasma and subsequent decreased blood volume may be followed by irreversible fluid loss in other ways such as diarrhea, vomiting, excessive sweating, burns, dehydration, and so on.

If the body is already dehydrated, this reaction will occur sooner. In places with high temperatures, such as warehouses and factories, or if the casualty sweats profusely before the injury (for example, accidents that occur while exercising or hunting) or some hard work, such as Bearing and forging may dehydrate the body before the accident, thus revealing the effects of reduced blood volume more quickly.

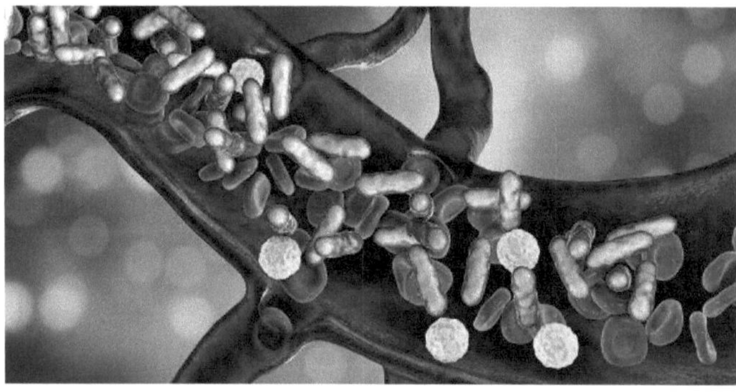

Figure 61. Septic Shock NCLEX Nursing Review Septic Shock NCLEX Nursing

Heart shock

Shock occurs if the heart is unable to pump blood properly and keep the body's arteries full of blood. The heart is a pump that pumps blood through the arteries into the body, and any abnormality in its output immediately manifests itself in reduced blood flow to various parts of the body. Cardiac output is a product of two factors:

Heart rate means the number of beats per minute.

Impact volume, that is, the volume of blood that leaves the heart during each beat.

Heart shock is usually caused by heart damage, heart attack and other heart diseases. Most heart disease that is delayed in treatment eventually causes so much damage to the heart that a heart attack occurs.

Shock caused by a change in the diameter of blood vessels

The capacity of the body's arteries should not be too large compared to the volume of blood. Dilation of blood vessels causes shock without sufficient contraction of other blood vessels (to compensate for this expansion). The body's arteries and veins can change their diameter in response to hormonal (chemical) and neurological effects. The sympathetic nervous system (part of the body's autonomic nervous system) is responsible for controlling the tension in the muscles in the walls of the arteries, and the activity of this system increases the contraction of the arteries. A similar effect is caused by hormones secreted by the adrenal glands, namely epinephrine and norepinephrine.

The contraction of the arteries significantly increases their resistance to blood. As a result, blood flow to the tissues decreases and at the same time arterial blood pressure increases. Conversely, decreased sympathetic activity leads to dilation of the arteries and increased blood flow to the tissues, while lowering blood pressure. In certain cases, when the blood vessels dilate too much, the blood pressure drops sharply and the casualty is shocked. Contraction of the veins can also cause high blood pressure by a different mechanism. At any given moment, most of the circulating blood volume in the veins causes a large volume of blood to move from the veins to the heart, which will increase blood pressure by increasing the output of the heart.

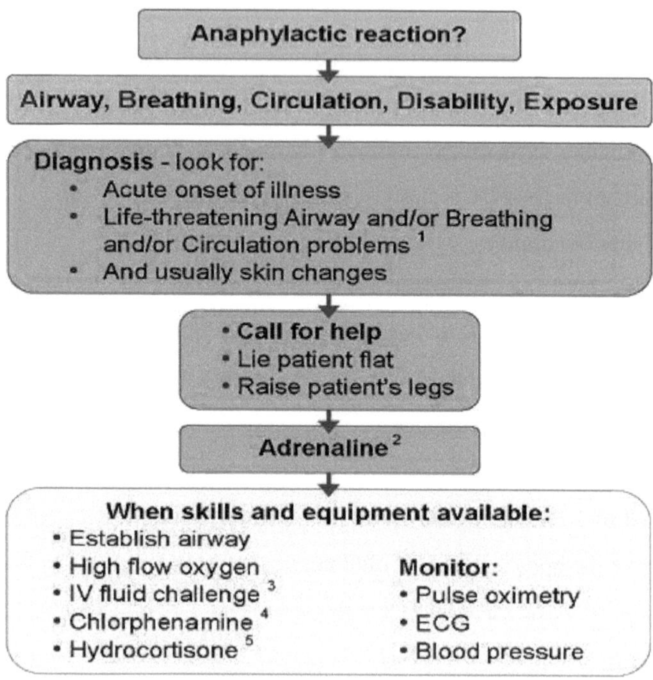

Figure 62. Anaphylactic Shock Case Study

Emergency measures in a patient with shock

The amount of time you have to take emergency measures for a person with a dangerous condition (severe bleeding and shock) is very short. Therefore, treatment should be started as soon as possible. Injured people who are shocked or at risk of shock should be rushed to a hospital.

Put the casualty in the right position Depending on the casualty's problems and injuries, he or she can be positioned:

Lifting the leg is the best way. Raise the injured leg 25 cm. Do not use this method in cases of injuries to the neck or spine, head injuries, chest and abdomen injuries, dislocations or fractures of the pelvis, or pelvic fractures. Do not place the casualty's body with his head and chest below body level, as this will cause the abdominal organs to press against the diaphragm. The goal is for the casualty to be in a position (open or half-sitting) that is completely comfortable and can breathe easily. In any situation you

put the casualty, you should check for vital signs and be careful because there is a possibility of vomiting.
Open the casualty's airway. To do this, place one hand on the injured forehead and the other hand under his chin. Bend the casualty's head back. This causes his mouth to open slightly. If the casualty is breathing, keep his or her airway open. If the casualty is not breathing, give artificial respiration. Watch out for secretions and vomit from the injured and wipe them off if present. If the casualty has stopped breathing and circulating blood, perform cardiopulmonary resuscitation (CPR). Control bleeding by applying direct pressure, holding the injured limb high, applying point pressure, or other necessary means. Decreased blood volume is dangerous for a shock victim. Wear shockproof clothing if available. If such a garment is not available, you can bandage the entire lower limb with medium pressure using bandages.
Deliver oxygen to the casualty as soon as possible. Lack of oxygen is caused by reduced blood flow. Provide pure oxygen to the casualty. Keep the casualty immobile if there is a possible injury to the spine.
Splint the fractures. This will reduce the bleeding and pain that both aggravate the shock. Do not shake the casualty sharply as the movement of the body intensifies the shock.
Reassure and strengthen the casualty and keep him or her still. If the injured are shocked, immobile and calm, they will have a better chance of surviving.
Avoid lowering body temperature. You should keep the casualty body temperature as close to normal as possible. But do not overheat the casualty. If possible, remove wet clothing from the injured person. Do not move injured people with head, spine, or neck injuries to place blankets under them.
Do not eat anything to the injured. The shocked person dries his mouth and feels thirsty. The victim's mouth and nasal passages may also become dry as a result of oxygen delivery to the casualty. The injured person should not drink anything. Do not give any medicine, food or liquid by mouth to the injured person. Doing so increases the risk of vomiting in the casualty.

The goal of primary treatment in volume shock is to prevent continued blood loss. Treatment is replacement of lost blood by giving fluid. In the first stage of treatment at the scene of the accident, a physiological serum (which is part of any relief equipment) or ringer lactate solution can be used. Ringerlactate solution contains salt in a concentration equal to the concentration of blood, and although it does not have blood cells and cannot perform all the functions of the blood, it can play an effective role in the early stages of replacement therapy and increase blood pressure. By doing this, lactate ringer helps maintain blood flow to all parts of the body. Blood transfusions are performed only with a doctor's prescription and during treatment.

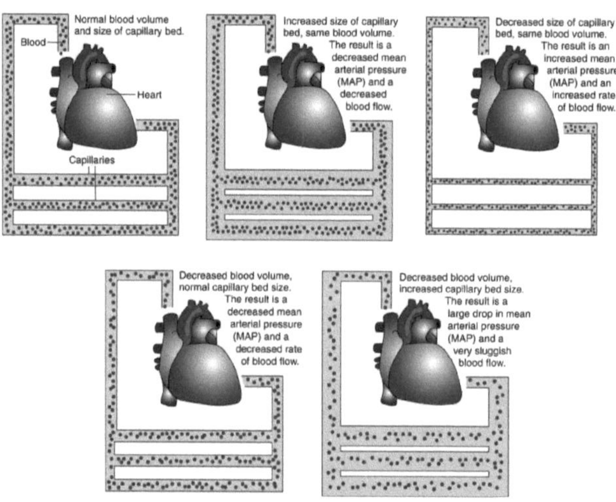

Figure 63. Care of Patients with Shock

Emergency measures in a patient with shock

The amount of time you have to take emergency measures for a person with a dangerous condition (severe bleeding and shock) is very short. Therefore, treatment should be started as soon as possible. Injured people who are shocked or at risk of shock should be rushed to a hospital.

Put the casualty in the right position Depending on the casualty's problems and injuries, he or she can be positioned:

Lifting the leg is the best way. Raise the injured leg 25 cm. Do not use this method in cases of injuries to the neck or spine, head injuries, chest and abdomen injuries, dislocations or fractures of the pelvis, or pelvic fractures. Do not place the casualty's body with his head and chest below body level, as this will cause the abdominal organs to press against the diaphragm. The goal is for the casualty to be in a position (open or half-sitting) that is completely comfortable and can breathe easily. In any situation you put the casualty, you should check for vital signs and be careful because there is a possibility of vomiting.

Open the casualty's airway. To do this, place one hand on the injured forehead and the other hand under his chin. Bend the casualty's head back. This causes his mouth to open slightly. If the casualty is breathing, keep his or her airway open. If the casualty is not breathing, give artificial respiration. Watch out for secretions and vomit from the injured and wipe them off if present. If the casualty has stopped breathing and circulating blood, perform cardiopulmonary resuscitation (CPR).

Control bleeding by applying direct pressure, holding the injured limb high, applying point pressure, or other necessary means. Decreased blood volume is dangerous for a shock victim. Wear shockproof clothing if available. If such a garment is not available, you can bandage the entire lower limb with medium pressure using bandages.

Deliver oxygen to the casualty as soon as possible. Lack of oxygen is caused by reduced blood flow. Provide pure oxygen to the casualty.

Keep the casualty immobile if there is a possible injury to the spine.

Splint the fractures. This will reduce the bleeding and pain that both aggravate the shock. Do not shake the casualty sharply as the movement of the body intensifies the shock.

Reassure and strengthen the casualty and keep him or her still. If the injured are shocked, immobile and calm, they will have a better chance of surviving.

Avoid lowering body temperature. You should keep the casualty body temperature as close to normal as possible. But do not overheat the casualty. If possible, remove wet clothing from the injured person. Do not move injured people with head, spine, or neck injuries to place blankets under them.

Do not eat anything to the injured. The shocked person dries his mouth and feels thirsty. The victim's mouth and nasal passages may also become dry as a result of oxygen delivery to the casualty. The injured person should not drink anything. Do not give any medicine, food or liquid by mouth to the injured person. Doing so increases the risk of vomiting in the casualty.

The goal of primary treatment in volume shock is to prevent continued blood loss. Treatment is replacement of lost blood by giving fluid. In the first stage of treatment at the scene of the accident, a physiological serum or solution of ringer lactate can be used. Ringer lactate solution contains salt in a concentration equal to the concentration of blood, and although it does not have blood cells and cannot perform all the functions of the blood, it can play an effective role in the early stages of replacement therapy and increase blood pressure. By doing this, ringer lactate helps maintain blood flow to all parts of the body. Blood transfusions are performed only with a doctor's prescription and during treatment.

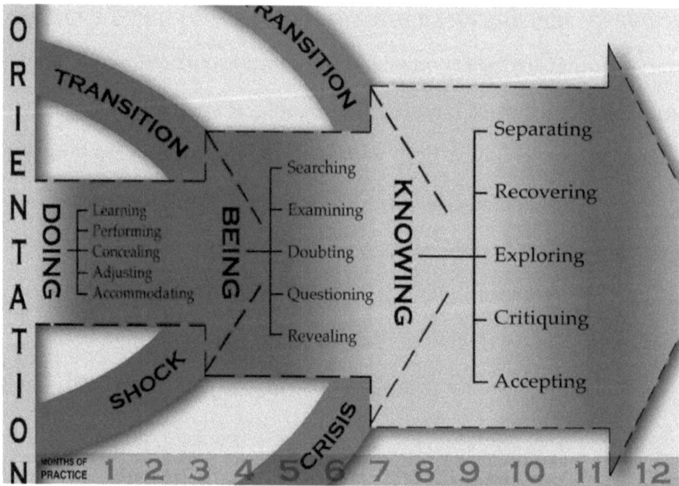

Figure 64. Contemporary nursing graduates' transition to practice

First aid (shock)

The circulatory system includes the heart as the pumping system of the blood vessels and blood vessels, whose job it is to deliver oxygenated blood and nutrients to the body's cells.

Definition

The reduction of vital signs of the body for various reasons immediately after injury or with a delay caused by the inability of the circulatory system to adequately deliver organs to the body is called shock, which varies from a weakness to a fatal condition due to severe injury. In this case, because not enough blood reaches the body, the body begins to cope with the current situation (reduced blood supply). In this case, the body's defense is such that maximum blood should reach the vital organs such as the brain and heart, while less important organs such as the skin, intestines and muscles should reach the blood, because the health of the heart and brain is more essential. It is against the reduction of blood supply.

This disorder can occur or progress for three reasons;

1- Decreased heart rate;
2- Sudden change in the diameter of blood vessels;
3- Insufficient volume of intravascular fluid.

Division of shock types

Shock due to decreased blood volume (hypovolemic) - Bleeding - Loss of fluids (non-bleeding such as diarrhea and vomiting)

Distributive shock - nervous shock

- Psychological shock (fainting)
- Infectious shock
- Anaphylactic shock

Heart Shock - Myocardial Infarction

Obstruction inside or outside the heart of blood circulation:

1- Shock of hypovolemia: Liquids make up 60% of the human body weight. Loss of 10% of this volume is compensated by compensatory mechanisms, but if the volume of circulating blood is reduced by 20-25%, the compensatory mechanisms are not able to compensate and hypovolemic shock occurs. This type of shock is one of the most common causes of shock, which can be caused by causes such as diarrhea, vomiting, profuse sweating, dehydration, internal and external bleeding, extensive burns, and acute events in the abdomen, such as rupture of the appendix.

2- Cardiac dysfunction shock (cardiogenic): The most common causes are diseases such as heart attack, heart injury, vascular hypertension in the lungs, aortic valve stenosis that 90-100% of patients die of heart attack.

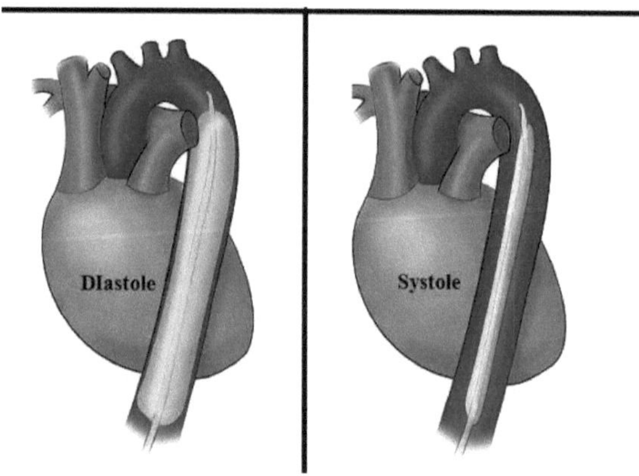

Figure 65. New Era of Intra-aortic Balloon Pump Market 2019-2023

3- Shock due to changes in vascular diameter (Vascular): In this shock, the blood flow to the tissues of the body is normal, but due to the secretion of chemical mediators that lead to impaired permeability and contraction of blood vessels, the volume of circulating blood seems low. This type of shock may occur due to the following factors:

A) Nerve shock (neurogenic): Spinal cord injuries cause a severe blow to the spine or head and cause pain and perception by the nervous system, and eventually a sudden dilation of blood vessels and a sharp drop in blood pressure.

B) Psychological shock (psychogenic): It is caused by a temporary and transient disturbance of blood flow to the brain for a few moments, such as hearing sudden news, extreme fatigue, standing for a long time, and so on.

C) Infectious shock (septic): The most common and important type of vasogenic shock is that pathogenic organisms cause this shock by releasing toxins in all tissues of the body by increasing the permeability of arteries and their dilation and dysfunction of the heart. Mortality from advanced infectious shock is high (about 50%), often due to severe hypotension and multiple organ failure.

D) Allergic shock (anaphylactic): In different stages of shock and types of shock such as infectious or allergic shock, the signs and symptoms are different, but in general, the signs of shock are:

- Pallor of the skin
- Cold and wet skin
- Rapid and weak pulse
- Rapid and shallow breathing
- Decreased blood pressure (late sign)
- Decreased body temperature
- Dilated pupils
- Nausea and vomiting
- Anxiety
- Restlessness
- Decreased level of consciousness or anesthesia
- Thirst
- Confusion

First Aid

The best treatment for shock is prevention. So if something happens to someone (for example, an accident) that you think is likely to cause a shock but still does not show signs of shock, still apply shock therapy to the person to avoid the shock.

These measures include:

I. Controlling and keeping the injured airways open and preventing aspiration of vomit.

II. Giving oxygen.

III. Bleeding control.

IV. Attaching the fracture site.

V. Lay the patient on his back and raise his legs about 20-30 cm. The important thing is to lower your legs immediately if this makes it difficult for the casualty to breathe, or do not raise the legs if there is a possibility of a broken leg or spine.

VI. Preventing the heat dissipation of the injured body by wrapping him in a blanket or quilt or anything similar, be careful not to heat the injured person with external heat (heater).

VII. If the casualty is not unconscious and does not vomit, give him fluids.

VIII. Control vital signs every 5 minutes.

Severe allergic reaction (anaphylactic shock)

Most people think that allergies only cause inflammation, itching, or other short-term problems that go away with eliminating the causative agent, but there are more severe reactions to certain foods or injections called anaphylactic shock. This shock can occur within minutes or even seconds and can be fatal if not treated immediately. Certain foods, such as nuts, oysters, fish, or certain medications, such as oral penicillin, bee or red bee stings, and injections of medications such as penicillin or tetanus vaccine, can cause severe and rapid reactions in sensitive people. About one percent of people are very sensitive to insect bites.

A severe allergic reaction (anaphylactic shock) occurs when a person comes into contact with an allergen and has a history of dealing with it and the body recognizes it as aggressive. In this case, an antibody called IgE is produced. The antibodies and host defenses then react with the allergen, which enters the body a second time, and chemicals (such as histamine) are released. These substances have unpleasant effects on the lungs, blood vessels, intestines and skin. This shock is one of the life threatening conditions. 60-80% of deaths due to anaphylactic shock are due to inability to breathe due to swelling and obstruction of the airways. The second cause of these deaths (about 24% of deaths) is shock, which is due to insufficient blood circulation.

Signs and symptoms of anaphylactic shock

- Cough, sneezing, wheezing Swelling of the face, tongue and mouth Difficulty breathing Nausea and vomiting Stiffness and swelling of the throat Dizziness.
- Severe itching and burning of the abdominal muscles (abdominal cramps).
- A rash or bluish skin rash (cyanosis) around the lips and mouth.
- In allergic shock, in addition to other shock first aid, adrenaline (epinephrine) is injected by the treatment team.

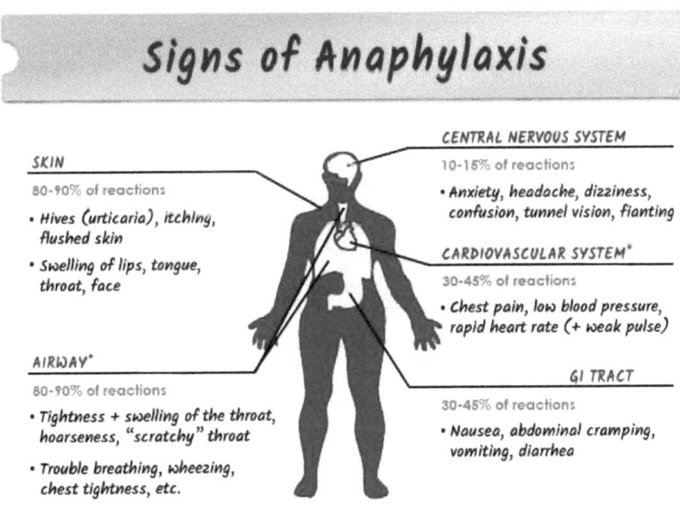

Figure 66. Anaphylaxis

Causes of allergic shock

Penicillin and its derivatives are the most common cause of anaphylactic shock, followed by snake bites, especially bee stings. The most common causes of anaphylactic shock are penicillin (and other drugs), foods (peanuts, eggs, seafood and milk), pollen extract, rubber and insect venom. Allergic shock is caused by the body's strong reaction to allergens and is very dangerous. Different types of substances can be allergenic.

For example, cat hair is allergenic. A person who is sensitive to cat hair will sneeze and itch whenever there is a cat near it. This reaction is very minor. In the case of bee stings, some people only react by feeling pain and swelling in the bee sting area. Some people also have more severe reactions or experience allergic shock. In this type of shock, the allergen causes the blood vessels to dilate rapidly and the blood pressure to drop. Also, the tissues in the airway become swollen and block the airways.

Allergens

Insect bites: Bee and red bee stings cause rapid and acute allergies.

Foods: such as fruits with oilseeds, spices, fruits such as (berry family), fish, oysters and some drugs, cause allergies. In most cases, this type of allergy is milder than insect bites.

Inhalants: Dust, pollen, and chemical powders often cause severe allergies.

Injectable: Drugs such as penicillin cause severe allergies.

Absorbents: Contact of certain chemicals with the skin of the body causes severe allergies. This type of shock cannot be accurately predicted.

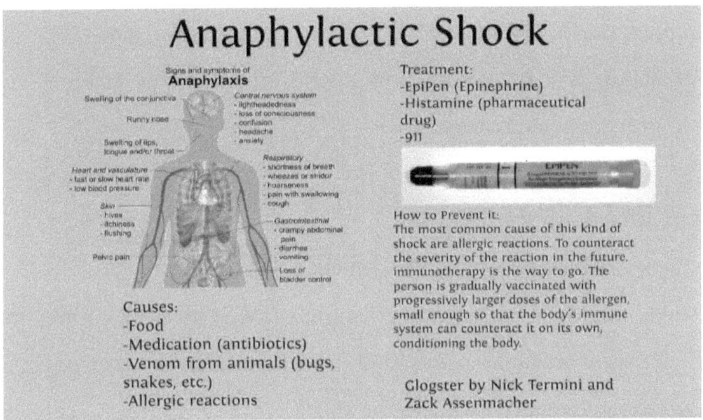

Figure 67. Emergency nursing, Nursing mnemonics, Anaphylactic shock

Symptoms of allergic shock

Level of consciousness: Restlessness, which is usually followed by fainting and anesthesia.

Breathing: It becomes difficult and is accompanied by wheezing.

Pulse: Beats fast and weak or is completely imperceptible.

Blood pressure: At first it is higher than normal, but it may later decrease to the point where it causes suspicion.

Skin: The effects of allergies are marked by redness and hives.

Face: Swelling of the tongue and face, bruised lips around the tongue and mouth become discolored.

Vomit

Swelling of the ankle and wrist

A patient with allergic shock usually complains of the following:

Itching and burning of the skin, especially the skin of the face, chest and back

Painful chest contractions and difficulty breathing

Vertigo

Restlessness and turmoil

Nausea, heartburn or diarrhea

Headache

Sneezing, itching, death, and hoarseness may be symptoms of shock.

This type of shock is a dangerous and urgent situation that requires injection of medication to prevent acute reactions.

Treatment of allergic shock

First of all, the sensitive agent must be identified and contacted.

Initial measures include Resuscitation Principles (BLS) measures. Open the patient's airway and perform artificial respiration or CPR. Deliver pure oxygen (in high concentration) to the casualty and treat the shock.

Take the casualty to a medical facility immediately. If the casualty is not unconscious, place him or her in an open or sideways position. Inform the medical staff if you are aware of an allergen or cause of allergies (e.g. insect bites, etc.). Perform the basics of resuscitation while transporting the casualty. Ask the casualty if he or she is allergic to a particular substance, including allergies to certain foods, environmental factors, certain medications, and other factors. Unknown factors are identified by the reaction shown by the casualty. Injured people who have a severe reaction to certain factors should take the necessary medication immediately if they come in contact with those agents.

The first injectable drug to treat allergic shock is the epinephrine ampoule, which is injected subcutaneously at a dose of about 0.01 mg / kg and up to a maximum of 0.3 mg. Subsequent medications include anti-allergic ampules such as chlorpheniramine, which are injected into a vein. Airway dilators such as aminophylline and immunomodulatory drugs such as hydrocortisone are also used. Intravenous fluid initiation, such as serum ringer lactate, is also important. Shock is caused by some relatively common childhood illnesses, including: gastroenteritis, diabetes mellitus, trauma, infection, and accidental ingestion of medication.

Note: The best clinical results of shock depend on early diagnosis and appropriate and prompt treatment. In infants, the myocardium has less contractile tissue, increasing the need for cardiac output, initially met by increasing the heart rate by neural mechanisms. In older children or adults, increasing the stroke volume very efficiently Increases the heart. Nursing attention in pediatric shock should focus on the cardiorespiratory and neurological systems. Changes in the level of consciousness are one of the first factors that indicate the worsening of the situation. Early diagnosis and prompt treatment of shock in infants and children reduces mortality. First of all, we must make sure that the airway is open and monitor the patient for breathing. It should also be ensured that the lungs open during respiration. Central blood flow is checked by checking the femoral, brachial, or carotid pulses.

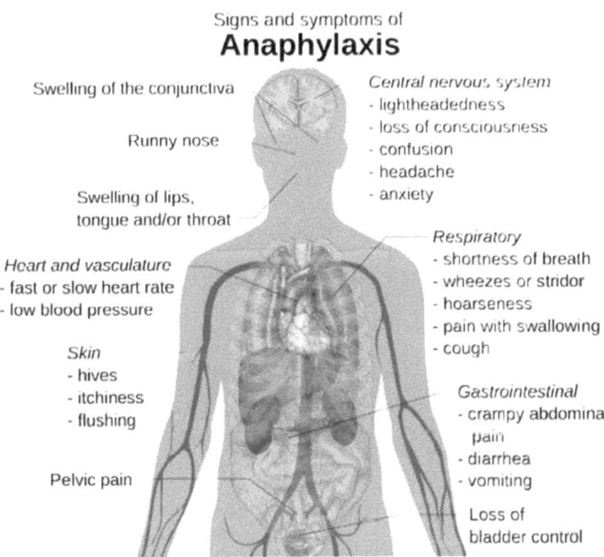

Figure 68. Anaphylactic Shock: A life-threatening reaction

Hypolic shock

The most common cause of shock in children and its causes are: loss of blood, loss of body fluids and electrolytes following vomiting and diarrhea, loss of fluid into the third space due to capillary leakage syndromes.

Hypolemic shock can be distinguished from other causes of shock by observing hypotension and tachycardia and the absence of symptoms of heart failure (such as hepatomegaly, rash, edema, jugular vein dilation or gallop) or toxic septum (fever, leukocytosis, or infection).

Improvement of hypolemic shock depends on the severity of the hypoplasia, the patient's heart condition, and rapid diagnosis and treatment. The prognosis of uncomplicated hypolemic shock is good and its mortality is less than 10%. Compensatory mechanisms in hypolemic shock include increased sympathetic and adrenal activity, which increases heart rate and myocardial contractility.
Children diagnosed with epileptic shock need to have vital signs checked, checking for BP every 15 to 60 minutes. Skin color and turgor, temperature should also be checked regularly. The anterior fontanelle should also be examined for indentation or protrusion. An indented fontanelle may be the cause of dehydration. On the other hand, the prominentness of the fontanelle usually indicates a sufficient level of body fluids. In addition, the nurse should regularly evaluate the patient's neurological symptoms. Decreased level of consciousness should be reported immediately. The nurse should regularly listen to the patient's heart and lungs and touch the peripheral pulses. Diarrhea. A bladder or Foley catheter should be used. The abdomen should be touched. Intestinal sounds should be heard. Abdominal injuries should be ruled out. Any injuries or trauma to the abdomen should be reported immediately.

Distributed shock (published)

Disorders of blood distribution may cause severe inadequate tissue blood supply, even if the output is normal or cardiac output is high. Septic shock is the most common distributive shock in children and is usually a complication of septicemia of gram-negative and gram-positive bacteria as well as infection caused by rickettsia and viruses. These patients usually have fever, drowsiness, and purpura, and an infection foci are found in their body. The initial sign of a distributed or diffuse shock is an increase in body temperature (hyperthermia) or a decrease in body temperature (hypothermia). The temperature should be checked every one to two hours. In premature shock (hyperdynamic phase) the skin usually becomes warm and shiny. In late shock (hypodynamic phase) the skin usually becomes cold and gray.

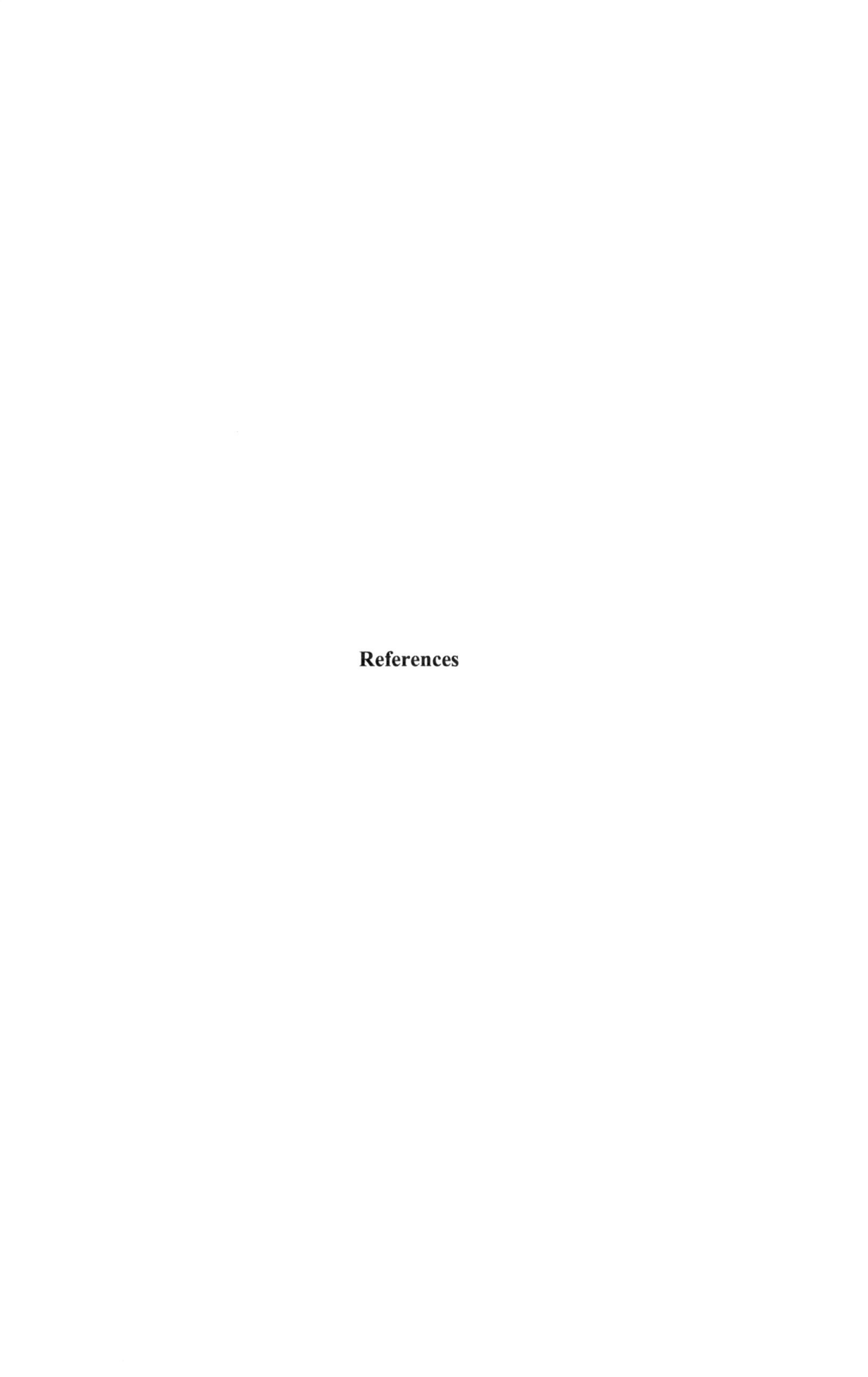

References

1. Kariman H, Heidarian A, Majidi A, Hatamabadi H, Dolatabadi AA, Azar BNF. Accuracy of inferior vena cava, aorta, and jugular vein ultrasonographic diameters in identifying pediatric dehydration. Iranian Journal of Emergency Medicine. 2015; 2 (4): 174 - 81.
2. Baratloo A, Rahmati F, Rouhipour A, Motamedi M, Gheytanchi E, Amini F, et al. Correlation of blood gas parameters with central venous pressure in patients with septic shock; a pilot study. Bulletin of emergency & trauma. 2014; 2 (2): 77.
3. Hall JE. Guyton and Hall textbook of medical physiology e- Book: Elsevier Health Sciences; 2010.
4. Hosenpud JD, Greenberg BH. Congestive heart failure: Lippincott Williams & Wilkins; 2007.
5. Goldman L, Ausiello D. Cecil Textbook of Medicine. 22nd ed2004. p. 669 - 76.
6. Brunicardi FC, Schwartz SI. Schwartz's principles of surgery. 8thed: McGraw- hill; 2005. p. 97 - 8.
7. Kasper D, Fauci A, Hauser S, Longo D, Jameson J, Loscalzo J. Harrison's principles of internal medicine, 19e. 16th ed2005. p. 1601- 6.
8. Downey DB. The retroperitoneum and great vessels. Diagnostic Ultrasound Philadelphia, PA, USA: Mosby, Inc. 3rd ed2003. p. 478- 80.
9. Alsous F, Khamiees M, DeGirolamo A, Amoateng- Adjepong Y, Manthous CA. Negative fluid balance predicts survival in patients with septic shock. Chest. 2000; 117 (6): 1749 - 54.
10. Salahuddin N, Chishti I, Siddiqui S. Determination of intravascular volume status in critically ill patients using portable chest X rays: measurement of the vascular pedicle width. Critical Care. 2007; 11 (2): P282.
11. Peachey T, Tang A, Baker EC, Pott J, Freund Y, Harris T. The assessment of circulating volume using inferior vena cava collapse index and carotid Doppler velocity time integral in healthy volunteers: a pilot study.

Scandinavian journal of trauma, resuscitation and emergency medicine. 2016; 24 (1): 108

12.Miller JB, Lee A, Suszanski JP, Tustian M, Corcoran JL, Moore S, et al. Challenge of intravascular volume assessment in acute ischemic stroke. The American journal of emergency medicine. 2018; 36 (6): 1018- 21.

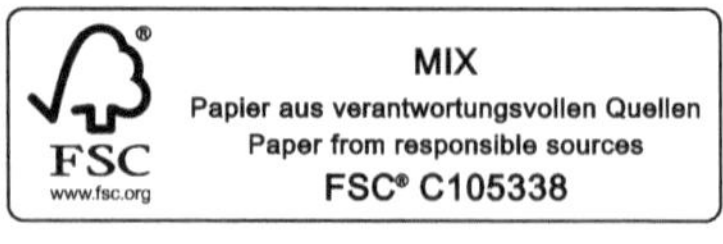

Printed by Books on Demand GmbH, Norderstedt / Germany